Happy Healing

8 Magic Steps to Relieve Physical Pain and Discomfort

Dominique Bourlet

Copyright © 2016 Bourlet House

All Rights Reserved. No part of this publication may be reproduced or transmitted in any form or by any means, mechanical or electronic, including photocopying and recording, or by any information storage and retrieval system, without permission in writing from the author or publisher (except by a reviewer, who may quote brief passages and/or show brief video clips in a review).

Disclaimer: The Publisher and the Author make no representation or warranties with respect to the accuracy or completeness of the contents of this work and specifically disclaim all warranties of fitness for a particular purpose. No warranty may be created or extended by sales or promotional materials. The advice and strategies contained herein may not be suitable for every situation. This work is sold with the understanding that the Publisher is not engaged in rendering legal, accounting or other professional services. If professional assistance is required, the services of a competent professional person should be sought. Neither the Publisher nor the Author shall be liable for damages arising therefrom. The fact that an organization or website is referred to in this work as citation and/or potential source of further information does not mean that the Author or the Publisher endorses the information, the organization or website may provide or recommendations it may make. Further, readers should be aware that internet websites listed in this work may have changed or disappeared between when this work was written and when it is read.

This book is not intended as a substitute for the medical advice of physicians. The reader should regularly consult a physician in matters relating to his/her health and particularly with respect to any symptoms that may require diagnosis or medical attention. The author and publisher advise readers to take full responsibility for their safety and know their limits. Before practicing the skills described in this book, be sure that your equipment is well maintained, and do not take risks beyond your level of experience, aptitude, training, and comfort level.

First Edition 2016

Printed in the United States of America

Published by:
Bourlet House
Winkler Strasse 16 B
Berlin, Germany, 14193

www.DomBourlet.com

For more information about Dominique Bourlet or to book him for your next event, speaking engagement, podcast or media interview please visit: www.DomBourlet.com

Table Of Contents

How To Read This Book

Happy Healing: 8 Magic Steps to Relieve Physical Pain and Discomfort is a book which will help you practice self-healing. Are you ready for Happy Healing?

HAPPY HEALING QUIZ

1. Is your physical and emotional well-being one of your priorities?

2. In particular, are you motivated by the perspective of staying pain free and of learning to start a healing process?

3. Do you believe that your emotions influence your physical health?

4. Would you be willing to be more in charge of your own health by applying a self healing protocol?

5. Are you interested by a new way to communicate with your body and its emotional intelligence?

6. Would you be willing to perform guided emotional work to improve your physical health?

7. Are you open to using innovative techniques to reduce pain?

8. Are you ready to heal yourself by loving yourself through an 8 step process?

If you answered "yes" to most of the questions, you are ready to learn more about how Happy Healing will improve your health and your life!

Reading for Specific Healing Goals

This section will help you to orientate your reading depending on your therapeutic priorities. I encourage you to read the entire book to learn all about Happy Healing; however, you may focus more intently on, or review, specific chapters.

Depending on your interests, goals, wishes, and needs, you may want to review the following chapters:

1. **Happy Healing in a nutshell**
   Read the Introduction, Happy Healing Visuals and Reporting Form (Chapter 6), Overview of the Method (Chapter 7), and The Three Prayers-Meditations (Chapter 8). Also read The Success Formula for Happy Healing and the Love Message (Chapter 17).

2. **The starting point of the method**
   Read the Introduction, Body Whispering (Chapter 2) and Speaking to the Body as a Person: The Story of Vendula (Chapter 3).

3. **Fixing quickly an acute pain**
   Read the Happy Healing Visuals and Reporting Form (Chapter 6), The Three Prayers-Meditations (Chapter 8), Case Studies and Your Health Issues (Chapter 12), and The Happy Healing Protocol (Chapter 15).

4. **Reducing a small discomfort**
   The task is more complicated than with an acute pain because the sensations are more subtle and more difficult to assess.

Read The Three Prayers-Meditations (Chapter 8), The Body Scan Procedure (Chapter 9), The Healing Equation of the Evaluation Process (Chapter 10), Case Studies and Your Health Issues (Chapter 12), The Happy Healing Protocol (Chapter 15), and The Success Formula for Happy Healing and the Love Message (Chapter 17).

5. **Just saying healing prayers and mantras**

   If you want to do simple emotional and spiritual work, without applying the whole healing protocol, just read The Three Prayers-Meditations (Chapter 8) and The Happy Healing Protocol, focusing on the healing mantras of the self-healing protocol, phase after phase, and the astral clapping out of gratitude (Chapter 15).

6. **Is Happy Healing particularly appropriate for a particular health issue?**

   Read The Benefits of Happy Healing (Chapter 4) and Case Studies and Your Health Issues (Chapter 12).

7. **Upgrading one's medical expertise with the self-healing initiative**

   Many patients wish to upgrade their medical and health expertise to practice self-healing and to be able to complement a specific medical treatment with emotional work.

   How to be more responsible, more in charge?

   Read The Sincere Wish to Heal (Chapter 1), Body Whispering (Chapter 2), and The Success Formula for Happy Healing and the Love Message (Chapter 17) to see how the philosophy of Happy Healing resonates with you: a philosophy of medical and health self-empowerment.

8. **Specific interest for new techniques related to body mind spirit themes**

   Read Speaking to the Body as a Person: The Story of Vendula (Chapter 3), The 12 Guidelines of the Happy Healing Process (Chapter 5), Happy Healing Visuals and Reporting Forms (Chapter 6), Overview of the Method (Chapter 7), The Three Prayers-Meditations (Chapter 8), The Body Scan Procedure (Chapter 9), The Tips of the Cosmos (Chapter 11), Happy Centering (Chapter 13), and The Happy Healing Protocol (Chapter 15).

9. **Seekers on the emotional and spiritual path**

   Read The 12 Guidelines of the Happy Healing Process (Chapter 5), The Three Prayers-Meditations (Chapter 8), The Tips of the Cosmos (Chapter 11), Happy Centering (Chapter 13), the Happy Healing Protocol (Chapter 15), and The Success Formula for Happy Healing and the Love Message (Chapter 17).

Introduction

Letting the Pain Go

Pain!
Suffering!
Very unpleasant indeed.

Strange creature, this Lady Pain. She comes and goes, but is never very far from us.

Lady Pain is like taxes. She reminds us of her presence a little too often, and we accept, more or less willingly, pain as a fact of life. Pain is also a tax on our happiness. Because of pain, we are less happy. Fortunately, tax havens exist.

This is what Happy Healing is about - no longer paying the tax on happiness thanks to emotional work that will set us free.

When Lady Pain comes, she brings not only unpleasant physical sensations, but also angst and fear of the future.

Lady Pain's message is alarming - something is going wrong with my body, and it could go from bad to worse! A little pain can increase and become chronic. The body's disbalance can be extended to other parts of the body. A snowball effect of pain, disease, and dysfunction could gain momentum. We have to take action!

What to do? Try to kill Lady Pain with painkillers? Remove the dysfunctioning body part with a surgical operation?

These approaches work well many times, but not always. They may create collateral damage because the body becomes a battle field in this military attempt to fight the pain and disease.

Happy Healing offers another way to neutralize Lady Pain. Rather than to try to kill Lady Pain, why not just open the door and let her go away, as peacefully as possible? Why not try to understand each other, discuss, and negotiate?

The Breakthrough

The breakthrough came for me in 2004. I had become an alternative practitioner in Europe after learning different manual therapies in Asia. My favorite tradition is Chinese acupressure. Medical acupressure is a powerful tool that is usually quite efficient. However, sometimes, without a clear reason, manual therapy is not tolerated by a patient.

Why? The truth of the matter appeared to me while treating a patient particularly upset with her own body: unconsciously, this patient did not emotionally support her Body-in-pain; instead, she perceived it as an enemy.

The mind thinks, "The pain comes from this part of my body. Therefore, this body part is producing pain and sending it to me. The Body-in-pain is my enemy. Not only I do not like it, but I am angry and frustrated towards it."

The higher the pain, the higher the negative feelings for the Body-in-pain. This leads to more difficulty in healing.

If somebody is experiencing a painful knee, he does not think, "Oh, my poor knee! I love you and I support you." Instead, he probably thinks, "My bloody knee is hurting me again!"

Every action creates an opposite reaction. This negative feeling is normal, legitimate, and explainable because of the pain. However, it will not help you heal.

On the contrary, the presence of a negative feeling for the Body-in-pain is the secret block that can prevent, or slow down, the healing process.

In a family, if a parent says to a child, "I do not love you, I hate you. Why did you come into my life? I wish you were never born," one can predict that the child will respond in many negative ways and the relationship will worsen.

When Lady Pain invites herself in, we resent our Body-in-pain. We are like the parents criticizing their child.

Therefore, it is a healing priority to remove this emotional block - the negative feeling towards the Body-in-pain.

The Happy Healing method was born from this intuition. Welcome to the community of the Happy Healers who benefit from this great mind-body medicine!

A New Method

Since this therapeutic intuition in 2004, I have treated hundreds of patients. Sometimes, it is one-on-one, other times, in small groups during workshops. In this book, I will show you how the Happy Healing method can be used as a method of self-healing without the help of a doctor or physical therapist.

To relieve physical pain thanks to emotional healing, however, there is a key prerequisite - we have to practice a soft approach, not a hard one.

I first realized the importance of a soft approach when learning about horse whispering. In *The Man Who Listens to Horses,* Monty Roberts describes this unique technique which uses gentle communication to create a partnership between horse and human. This same positive communication can help patients form a healing relationship with their Bodies-in-pain.

In the Happy Healing process, the Body-in-pain is considered a person, a suffering being gifted with emotional intelligence. When you use the Happy Healing protocol, you will be given the opportunity to determine the gender and traits of your Body-in-pain. Within this text, the patient will be presented as feminine and the Body-in-pain will be considered masculine.

The Magic Steps of Happy Healing

In eight magic steps, the Happy Healing Protocol proposes a soft approach to tame the unconscious mind, to tame our negative feelings towards the body. By doing so, the pain will be released without fighting the Body-in-pain. Elegant, fast, gentle, and so efficient!

Happy Healing starts with an **evaluation** in two phases (A and B). It then organizes the **transformation** of the feelings for the body in two cycles.

In **Phase A**, a **body scan** will be performed to examine which parts of the body are in pain or discomfort and with what intensity.

In **Phase B**, a **name** will be given to the body part in pain, and **the negative feelings for the body will be identified.**

In the first cycle of **3 phases (1 to 3), the negative feelings will be decreased,** slowly, but surely.

In the second cycle of **3 phases (4 to 6), the positive feelings will be increased** progressively.

During this emotional transformation, thanks to the Mind Mood Management of Happy Healing, positive emotions corresponding to a succession of positive visualizations will flush out the negative feelings and build up the positive feelings. Physical pain and discomfort will be released along the way, while the healing process gains momentum.

Isn't it wonderful? Happy Healing brings not only pain relief, but also happiness. You'll feel a new set of positive emotions towards your body.

- In PART ONE, the creation of the method will be reviewed.
- PART TWO will offer a detailed description of Happy Healing.
- Finally, in PART THREE, you will discover the 8 magic steps of the self-healing protocol.

As you begin to use Happy Healing, you may want to start
by using the much shorter 4 step version of the protocol.
It is a wonderful way to familiarize yourself with
the protocol and your own healing.

Visit **www.HappyHealingBook.com/bonus**
to receive your copy of this bonus mini-protocol.

Best wishes for this journey to the land of Happy Healing, to the realm of physical, emotional, mental, and spiritual well-being!

PART ONE

The Creation Of The Method

*"A gentle approach
which honors the body spiritually,
cherishes him emotionally
and takes care of his physical integrity"*

— Chapter 2, Body Whispering

CHAPTER 1

The Sincere Wish To Heal

When Lady Pain knocks on the door, it is not good news. Nobody wants to let Lady Pain in. Too late: Lady Pain is already inside and making herself at home. Normally, everyone would like her to leave as soon as possible.

However, Lady Pain knows her job. She knows how to stay, and how to be tolerated, and then accepted. She brings a few advantages. She becomes a companion. A demanding companion, but a companion.

Let us review some of those advantages.

If the patient leads a monotonous life, disease and pain bring adventure and a form of excitement, even if the context may be highly alarming. Pain spices up life. The thrill of the pain drama counterbalances the "tax on happiness" and makes it bearable.

In some occasions, disease is the only way for a patient to escape exhausting obligations or life situations. A "burn out" is the unconscious way to say no to an excessive workload and to take a break. The body, when pushed beyond a certain limit, refuses to operate like before and goes on strike.

This is the infinite wisdom of the body. Pain and disease are warning signals indicating that something is wrong at some level. Lady Pain is saying, "Stop! Think! Time to Change and Adjust!"

Disease is also one way for some patients to influence their relatives and friends to help them, to visit them more often, to support them, and to listen to them. It is one way to gain attention and sympathy. We all need to be loved. To stimulate compassion of others, disease is sometimes the magic tool. Of course, it has a cost. However, the benefit of becoming the center of the attention and having a moving story to tell is not to be discounted.

There is a form of pride in acting in the very special scenario of illness. Some patients mention the long and complicated medical name of their disease with the satisfaction of a collector showing a great piece of artwork.

Of course, disease and pain are many times a tragedy, having an impact on a whole family or community. However, one can get used to it, and then, resignation will perpetuate the tragedy.

Many patients get trapped in a state of unfortunate resignation to sickness and pain.

How to get out? Difficult, when the patient feels she has no energy, time, or money to look for an appropriate treatment and follow it. These three handicaps, in the perception of the patient, are sometimes combined. The end result is resignation.

The patient establishes herself in an uncomfortable comfort zone. A second best situation that she learns to live with. Insidiously, disease and pain become long-term residents.

The patient becomes discouraged or skeptical about finding the right healing solution.

She has consulted doctors, undertaken various medical examinations and tests, tried different medications, but seen no real improvement.

She thinks, "If doctors who studied 7 years and more, equipped with top technology, cannot find an effective therapy for me, then, at my level, without such a medical training and experience, how can I alone find a solution? My situation is hopeless."

Patients learn to suffer and repress their pain or discomfort. Sometimes, when I ask somebody apparently in pain if she is in pain, the answer is, "Not too bad; it is okay." When I ask this person to grade the sensation between 0 and 10, the answer is often a 5 or even more.

This means people under the attack of pain, sometimes chronic pain, become more and more resilient in one way, and accept higher levels of pain without even noticing it. The patient adjusts to the painful situation and accepts it because she feels she has no choice. The danger is resignation. Instead of taking action, procrastination.

In this resignation process, if the patient "capitulates" and does not take action for her main painful spot, she will very likely ignore other spots of pain or discomfort. Resignation is taking over. The messages of the body are not paid attention to.

The trouble with this attitude is that the higher the pain level is allowed to go, the higher the risk of further complications, of an extension of the number of painful spots. The horizon seems blocked. What to do?

Cultivate a more positive attitude. Do not lose hope. Wish sincerely to heal and start practicing self-healing!

Positive Energy

In this regard, one of the best lessons I learned was in Thailand.

In a few years, I learned more than 20 massage protocols in all Asia, from India to Japan, in at least 10 Asian countries with well-rooted therapeutic traditions.

The school which impressed me the most is the Wat Pho School in Bangkok.[1] This school of Thai Yoga Massage offers various courses of 5 days, 6 hours a day.

---

[1]   "Watpo Thai Traditional Massage School." 2003. <http://www.watpomassage.com/>

What is incredible is that students, complete beginners or advanced therapists, can join any day, morning or afternoon, all year round, except two days per year! There is maximum flexibility. Students arrive, they are integrated into a course with five other students, at the most, by a smiling teacher. After a few minutes of explanations, they are invited to practice hands on with other students lying on a mat.

No administrative complications, no big theoretical presentations, no complex anatomical, physiological or pathological descriptions. Hands on, with the motivation to do well and to rejuvenate the energy of the student lying on the mat by applying centuries old basic gestures of Thai massage.

Immediately, the new student feels accepted and participates to the transmission of this wonderful massage tradition, so popular now, not only in Thailand, but in many parts of the world. I found great joy in bringing a new energy to students lying on the mat, and afterwards, experiencing in turn this magic energy released by Thai massage, close to the monumental statues of Lord Buddha in the Wat Pho Temple.

How is it possible to alleviate human suffering? This is the central question of Buddhism. The Wat Pho School shows the way, pragmatically, simply, in a very efficient and relaxed way. A showcase for a positive healing attitude.

I must say that I have a great gratitude for this school, not only for the great teachings, but also for this introduction to practical Buddhism, a philosophy of practical self-healing.

Self Empowerment through Self-healing

The danger with sophisticated medical technology is that patients search endlessly for the physical cause of their health issues.

Instead of focusing on a self-healing approach, patients are depending on medical tests and examinations. No, it is not because the patients are investing time and money in a detailed search for diagnosis that the cure has started. It could lead, on the contrary, to a depressed state of mind because this material investigation does not always give clear directions.

Rather than worrying so much, the patient should focus on the small positive steps bringing relief and relaxation on the physical and psychic level.

Massage, manual therapy, is one of these positive solutions that is always good to practice with the appropriate touch depending on the health issues.

Happy Healing is another solution, an emotional healing solution, fully in line with the Wat Pho spirit of Buddhist pragmatism: if you are in pain, try to reduce it, even if you do not know the exact cause of this pain. If you can reduce it empirically, isn't it wonderful?

The great hope that Happy Healing is bringing to a suffering patient can be formulated like this:

You are suffering. Let us use all the painful sensations of your body as a tool that will help you to control the situation and to reverse the illness process.

You, and only you, are the #1 best expert in the world on your pain and discomfort. If you deepen your expertise, you can launch a very successful self-healing initiative.

I suppose that the patient is rightfully proud of herself! Sometimes the truth is well hidden, but very close, here, within the body. Let us continue this dialogue with the spirit of Happy Healing:

Inside your body, you experience many pleasant and unpleasant physical sensations. These unpleasant sensations bring physical discomfort, which is usually painful, but not always.

These sensations are symptoms for health issues. Symptoms that are not only clinical, like a medical test, but symptoms that you experience in your body, the intensity of which you can grade between 0 and 10. Very important: you are "living" these symptoms, you are feeling them concretely. Let us call them "SENTIOMS," like "sentient" symptoms.

Once again, you are the #1 best expert in the world to know what you are really experiencing hour after hour, minute after minute. No machine, no wonder doctor can experience as well as you your sensations, symptoms, and sentioms.

With the body scan practiced in phase A of Happy Healing, you will learn to note down all these sentioms and qualify them.

They are very important. They are not only material information; they are the very messages of your Body-in-pain, which wants to communicate with you. They are the screams and tears, the sighs and whispers of your suffering body, which does not only want to TALK TO YOU with these warning signals, but also wants to talk WITH YOU and have YOU TALK BACK.

If you want to help your body out of pain and sickness, you must welcome all these unpleasant sensations with a sense of detachment and with an acute attention or mindfulness, in line with Buddhist philosophy.

Once you become just the observer of your sensations or sentioms, without an on-going frustration or resentment, then you can start transforming them with the Happy Healing Protocol.

Sensations come and go; emotions and feelings come and go. After the first phase, when you observe your sensations and feelings with neutrality instead of a confused impression of wild and unjustified suffering, then you can enter a phase of sympathy and later on, of love, which will definitely start reducing the unpleasant sensations.

Be full of hope: try this new positive observation of your sensations many times. Get to understand this language of your Body-in-pain. Be satisfied with impressive results, but also with very small results. What is important is to go in the right direction. Feel grateful for every little positive move!

This self-healing initiative is accessible to every patient who wishes sincerely to heal and to apply the Happy Healing Protocol.

To take immediate action, do not wait for a high level of pain. The quicker you address your health issue, the easier it will be to regulate and the less unpleasant your illness experience will be. This is the huge advantage of early prevention. Physical health prevention and maintenance starts with the emotional "maintenance" of positive emotions.

RECOMMENDATION #1: As soon as you feel a painful or uncomfortable spot, complete the body scan procedure, and go through the Happy Healing process.

Be in charge, be your own expert, and take action, even with small warning signals. Your health is your business, the result of the communication between your Body-in-pain and you. To be in good health, learn to answer the messages of your body.

Practice with self-confidence the health self-empowerment of Happy Healing.

Honor your body, respect him, and love him, even if it is hard at the beginning. Speak with him! Then, you will be guided to a recovery.

CHAPTER 2

Body Whispering

Why try to obtain by force that which can be obtained through gentle negotiation? This is the whole concept of Happy Healing.

In order to facilitate the creation of a positive mindset for a treatment, the ideal patient should first receive an education, or more exactly, a re-education, concerning the basic notions of pain, symptoms, disease, and the Body-in-pain.

Each term may be viewed as a coin with two faces. No need to just present the negative aspects of the dark face, the unpleasant and frightening ones. It is important to perceive fully the positive aspects of the other face, the bright face.

Pain

Pain is a warning signal. The body gives a few hints. If they are not perceived, or perceived and not understood, or understood but ignored, the next level is pain. The nervous system is an alarm system. Beware! The lights are blinking: this is what pain wants to say.

Nature wants to protect us. The alarm system is part of a protection mechanism.

We should, therefore, be admirative and grateful when the alarm system is working. A burglar is working in our body. Rather than complaining about the noisy alarm, which is disturbing our quietness, we should be grateful and investigate why a burglar broke in and what he wants to steal from us.

Pain is an ally of the body, not an enemy. A special ally, it is true, a disturbing ally, but fundamentally, an ally.

The positive voice inside ourselves could say, "Welcome, pain, good that you came in, good that you are here. Thanks to you, I will take care of my body. Without you, I would continue to overload my body with tasks that he can no longer perform."

The Happy Healing attitude starts with challenging the perception that pain is unpleasant; alternatively, it plays a positive role in maintaining our body. Paradoxically, we could say: "Hello, Happy Pain!"

Symptoms

Symptoms are also warning signals. Though they might be not as unpleasant, they remain important messages of distress and need to be properly deciphered. Then, action is needed to take away the causes that produced the symptoms.

Disease & Sickness

Pain and symptoms are often accompanied by sickness or disease, which also convey a positive meaning beyond the unpleasant experience. Disease can be viewed as an adjustment process, a reaction to eliminate, to purify, to detoxify.

Fever has its virtues; its role is to "burn" bad germs. An abscess concentrates toxins and release them after an inflammation phase.

If these adjustments are manifesting themselves too strongly, it is sometimes necessary to curb them. However, we must not interfere unduly and hinder Mother Nature from doing natural, healthy adjustments.

Many symptoms are wrongly considered diseases. High blood pressure, for example, is not a disease; it is the indication that the heart, this complex muscle, is over exerting itself. Like with pain, we must learn to view more positively the role of disease when it occurs.

Another important way to look at disease, this bio-shock for the body, is to measure the opportunities that disease presents.

If the patient is overcoming, in the right way, the challenge of the disease, sometimes terrible and life threatening, she can gain strength and spiritual growth from this trial.

So many cancer survivors illustrate this powerful transformation achieved during the healing process. New sets of values, essential re-centering, heart opening, less worrying, especially over small details, more positive emotions: a long list of achievements rewards the happy challengers.

Disease shuffles the cards. New orientations appear. Disease pushes people to react, to mobilize all their forces on many levels, to shake the old routine and to re-invent themselves. Disease is sometimes a unique opportunity for a new birth, a new start in life.

When disease announces herself, let us greet the challenge and make the best out of it.

If we can integrate this positive view of pain and disease, we are building up a very sound basis to unleash the Happy Healing Process.

Body-In-Pain

You have already learned that a major block for healing is the unconscious perception by any patient in pain that, since the body is sending pain, he is therefore the culprit and the enemy.

Happy Healing is an emotional process to erase this perception and to substitute the opposite perception: the suffering body is not the worst enemy, but the patient's best friend!

Upstream, it is good to already deprogram the usual negative views on pain and disease, and to emphasize the importance of a positive attitude.

If pain and disease are considered to be dangerous enemies, what happens? The risk is that the treatment that will be chosen and the way it will be implemented will be a little too aggressive and invasive.

If "war" is declared against disease, if we try to "kill" pain with "painkillers," the big issue is that the body might become the battle field of this military fight, the collateral victim of a heavy and massive treatment.

In the end, it happens that patients sometimes heal from the disease, but die of exhaustion, with an immune system totally weakened by the military-like medical campaign fought too vigorously.

Between the resignation and the procrastination on one hand, and an aggressive and invasive treatment, is it not possible to opt for a third path, the middle path of the soft attitude?

So many fine tunings to do in the first place: detoxifying the body (intestines, gall bladder, kidneys, blood), reinforcing the immune system, increasing the energy level (thanks to energy massages), practicing flexibility exercises to relax the tense zones of the body, breathing exercises, mental concentration with meditation, transmuting negative emotions into positive ones as Happy Healing is advocating…

Then, if necessary, a more powerful and invasive approach can be implemented, including surgery. But why not try at the beginning **a gentle approach which honors the body spiritually, cherishes him emotionally and takes care of his physical integrity?**

To anchor this attitude, we must reframe our perception of the usual medical concepts such as pain and disease. Then loving the Body-in-pain, this so powerful key for quick and sustainable healing, will seem not only fine and beautiful, but also obvious and elementary for practical results.

This is the great goal of Happy Healing: treating the Body-in-pain as a partner who needs, sometimes desperately, our full emotional support.

We could call this attitude "BODY WHISPERING" in the same way as this new generation of Californian horse trainers are now called "horse whisperers" and no longer "horse breakers."

Why this reference to whispers? It is said that for spectators of this new horseman's practice, the horseman seemed to "whisper" to his horse's ears, who then complied with what was requested from him.

In 1998, in the Czech Republic, I gave many workshops to present this soft approach practiced in California. It enables a horse rider to gently persuade a young horse to be saddled for the first time. The process usually takes place in less than one hour in a round pen.

A revolution in the world of horse riding! Normally, the process of "breaking" or taming a horse lasts approximately two months and may be dangerous for the rider and the horse, because of the violence which may occur.

The comparison is clear - the soft approach of horse whispering is fast, fairly peaceful, efficient, and creates a good bond between the rider and the horse. The old way of horse "breaking" is a harder approach, which takes a lot of time, can be dangerous, and can traumatize the young horse.

It seems that the soft approach is preferable. However, it requests a gentle touch, an emotional openness to understand the horse's psychology and to speak with him.

Likewise, if we leave the horse world to come back to the health world, to reduce the pain, we have the choice between these two options: the soft one and the tough one.

Healing can be much easier to unleash if we proceed with the right emotional attitude, the soft and gentle attitude.

Happy Healing could be defined as a "body whispering" method. To reduce the pain, no violence, no attempt to "break" the Body-in-pain to subdue him. The strategy consists in taming a very special wild horse. This rebellious mustang is…the unconscious mind of the patient!

Yes, if we learn to change our unconscious mental attitude towards the Body-in-pain, we will change our feelings for the body, and we can heal.

When the body sends light pain signals, subtle discomforts, it is as if the body was "whispering" his distress to the patient. Reversely, when the patient is practicing a soft therapeutic approach, it is as if she was "whispering" her understanding of the situation to the body, and sending subtle energetic help to him.

Let us compare again horse training and therapy, horse whispering and now "body whispering." In both cases, the idea is to "tame" the mind, the wild unconscious mind: the mind of the horse reluctant to the proposed training, the mind of the patient reluctant to heal or reluctant to involve herself in a specific therapy.

How to Address Avoidance Tactics

As a horse whisperer 18 years ago, I learned quickly to evaluate the attitudes of the horses brought to me in a round pen for the first saddling session of their life.

I have done a certain number of workshops in public, and I had to meet the expectations of the spectators - in less than one hour convince the young horse to accept saddle and rider on his back. I could not say to the audience, "Come back next week, the horse is not ready today." I had to show that the horse whispering method was working, whatever the reaction of the horse.

After a few seconds, I could classify the horses coming in the round pen, or arena, in four categories: aggressive horses (usually stallions), defensive horses (usually mares), unfocused horses (usually castrated horses or geldings), or fearful horses and mares.

For each category, I had a different proven strategy. Always a soft attitude, trying to understand the animal, and matching his psychology.

With aggressive stallions, I avoided dominant gestures and tried to act firmly, but softly. I had to make clear to the stallion that I was not interested in a fight with him, but wanted to come to a gentle agreement.

With defensive mares, I had to persevere and insist, gently but surely, to make them understand that I would be gentle, but that I would not give up.

With unfocused horses, I had to enter their personal space in a more invasive way so that they understood that we had to enter into a partnership together and that they had to interact with me.

With the fearful horses and mares, I needed to make myself transparent, not threatening in the least, apparently not interested by any interaction with them. Then when the fearful horses became curious and intrigued, I could start an interaction with them with a very soft approach.

In all four cases, the horse whispering soft approach was modulated according to the horse's basic behavior.

These four categories apply also to the therapist-patient relationship. How to convince the unconscious mind of a patient to accept in a spirit of cooperation, not the saddle, but the best healing treatment?

In self-healing, the patient is, at the same time, the patient and her own therapist. Her main task is also to be sure on an unconscious level that she has a sincere wish to heal, and that she is ready for the middle path between resignation and aggressive treatment.

The aggressive stallion stands for the patient who will rush into the treatment without kindness for her body, in a materialistic way. For such a patient, the body is a machine, and needs no emotional support.

The defensive mare represents the patient who will accept initially a treatment, but suddenly will wish to step out, and will refuse to go further.

The unfocused horse is the patient who will "zap" between different treatments, and who will be superficially committed, unable to really start a treatment with the necessary commitment which will bring healing success.

Last category, the fearful horse is another type of challenge: the patient fears to leave her "uncomfortable comfort zone," and therefore, refuses to experiment a treatment which could harm her or generate negative changes if not appropriate. Such a patient is also afraid of entering an emotional process. Her emotions are buried deep inside, and the thought of letting the emotions go out this secret hideaway makes her too anxious.

The good therapist will quickly understand what type of patient is in front of him. His mission is not only to find the right therapy but also to "sell" this therapy to the patient's unconscious mind, to persuade her gently that the therapy is good for her, and to motivate her to take a healing commitment. This is perhaps the highest skill of the therapist.

The good horse whisperer will, in a sort of interspecies telepathy, convince the young horse to accept quickly, and in a spirit of harmony, a training to the saddle, to avoid a fight mutually detrimental. Likewise, the therapist helps the patient to nurture the best healing attitude as possible.

The patient will then honor her body, and treat him with respect and kindness and perseverance to welcome and trigger the healing.

RECOMMENDATION #2: Consider Pain as a messenger and an instrument and your Body-in-pain as a friend, not as an enemy, a friend who is weakened and who needs your full support, not your judgment and critics, and who needs from you love and not frustration and resentment.

Then tame your unconscious mind and be sure that you are nurturing the right healing attitude. Neither resignation, nor aggressiveness towards the Body-in-pain, but a patient, subtle and loving body whispering. A good self-healer is a good body whisperer.

Speaking To The Body As A Person: The Story Of Vendula

We have seen the importance of the right healing attitude to practice self-healing and, in particular, to apply the Happy Healing Protocol. I will now explain how the basic ideas of Happy Healing came to my mind twelve years ago in central Europe.

I had given a medical acupressure session to a female patient whose uterus was sometimes bleeding excessively. The relaxing treatment was well received and the patient felt relieved. She expressed the wish to come back for another session. However, when she came back a week later, her attitude had changed and she seemed embarrassed. I became intrigued: the reaction to the treatment had been positive…what could be the problem?

The patient explained that her gynecologist was ready to operate to remove her uterus. A routine operation, according to her, without any consequence since she was over forty and did not wish to have any more children.

I expressed a different view, explaining that the uterus was an important organ. After its removal, the syndrome of the phantom missing organ could manifest itself. Perhaps a manual therapy treatment could help the uterus to function without hemorrhage? Then the huge bio-shock of the surgical operation, the so-called "hysterectomy," an awe-inspiring word, with the risk of altering the organic balance achieved by Mother Nature, could be perhaps avoided. At least, it was worth trying a manual treatment a few more weeks.

I felt the strong opposition of my patient, as if she had fallen under a spell which made her incapable of listening to my logical arguments. What could I do? To test the state of mind of my patient, I had suddenly an intuition, which, I hoped, would be a life saving intuition. I knew I only had a few seconds to find a way to plead for the cause of the uterus and a few minutes to present my pleading.

I felt very tense. I had met a few women in an Ayurvedic clinic in north India whose uterus had been saved thanks to a proper diet and a special oil treatment. I could not propose an identical treatment; however, my duty was to persuade this patient to reconsider her position.

In a few microseconds, I felt a great compassion for the uterus of this woman, and of all women.

In Sanskrit, the traditional language of India, uterus is "yoni." The female communities can consider themselves part of the "Yoniversum," the "Yoni-universe."[2] The uterus is the sacred link between women and men. Without a uterus, human beings could not be conceived and could not be given birth to.

I was feeling concerned, not only as a therapist, but also as a human being. I heard myself saying, "Could you give a name to your uterus? Yes, a name, as if your uterus were a person, a person with a soul?"

The question was crazy, but I felt compelled to ask it as it came. The patient replied quickly in a cold tone, "VENDULA."

"And what is your feeling towards VENDULA?" I asked back…

The answer was prompt, "I hate her, I hate VENDULA."

---

[2]   Camphausen, Christina. "Yoni in Sanskrit." *The Yoniverse.*
<http://yoniversum.nl/yoni/define.html>

The situation was now clear. Dissimulating my stupefaction, I tried to plead in favor of VENDULA...Why not try some more manual treatment, other therapies, changing diet, before the removal operation? Why such a strong feeling against VENDULA? Could my patient send some sympathy to her uterus, such an important organ for a woman?

My attempt was utterly rejected. After a small conversation, the lady summarized her position in a way which was final. "I understand what you are saying...I do believe that if I could have some sympathy for VENDULA, I could receive other acupressure treatments...the surgical operation could be probably postponed and perhaps avoided...but I will tell you the truth, my deep truth: I have no sympathy whatsoever for VENDULA, and I do not want to have any sympathy for her...If you knew how I hate VENDULA!

This hatred is so strong that I want to stay with it. In one way, I like it and I need it...I know it sounds weird...I prefer to lose my uterus rather than attempt to show VENDULA, of course not love, but even some sympathy...Thank you for your first treatment which was pleasant and brought me some relief. But I have made my decision...I will not come back. I will do the surgical operation."

Two months later, I learned from a common friend that the patient had the operation. Gone was her uterus and ovaries.

Of course, I respected the decision of this patient. But this sad story had the merit to give me a powerful therapeutic intuition: a patient can personify the Body-in-pain by creating a name and a description for this person, gifted with an emotional intelligence. Then the EGO, the "I" of the patient could express his subconscious feelings towards the Body-in-pain, which were negative because of the distortion of pain.

This moving story was my epiphany for Happy Healing.

Thanks to this encounter with Vendula, I discovered the importance of the emotional attitude of the patient towards the Body-in-pain, the sick, suffering body.

I had received 4 major teachings.

- The first teaching was that the Body-in-pain is perceived unconsciously and sometimes consciously by the patient as an enemy producing and sending pain.
- The second teaching is a consequence: the irritation of the Ego is so high sometimes that a surgical removal of the Body Part in pain is viewed subconsciously not only as a medical necessity, but also as a revenge against the troublemaker, a death punishment which eliminates the enemy forever.
- The third teaching is that by giving a name to the Body Part in pain, the patient can face the body as a person, and evaluate her feelings for this person, feelings which are negative, and sometimes highly negative, not only preventing healing and the wish to heal, but also favoring the surgical removal.
- The fourth teaching was the vision that naming the Body-in-pain and starting to talk positively with the Body-in-pain as a person gifted with his own emotional intelligence was a good way to recreate the love flow for the body, which is the life flow. The Happy Healing protocol was born!

Practicing Happy Healing is like the re-enactment of the Vendula story, but this time, like in the family constellations therapy[3], rewriting the story with a happy ending.

---

[3]   "Family Constellation - Bert Hellinger offizielle Homepage ..." 2010. <http://www2.hellinger.com/en/home/family-constellation/>

RECOMMENDATION #3: Consider your body as a person, a being gifted with an emotional intelligence. Give him a name and speak with him. You will be able to observe your feelings for him, usually negative if your body is in pain.

Then you will be able to decrease your initial frustration and love your body progressively. You will not only enjoy a wonderful emotional moment, you will also heal your body and relieve the pain and discomforts which are disturbing both him and you.

CHAPTER 4

The Benefits Of Happy Healing

Highly negative feelings for the Body-in-pain block the wish to search for a proper treatment and heal. This was Vendula's lesson.

Conversely, the ambition of Happy Healing is to foster highly positive feelings for the Body to trigger the wish to heal and the self-healing forces.

One of the first applications of the Happy Healing protocol that I made was for patients who could not tolerate any physical touch, or only a very light pressure. Quite embarrassing for a manual therapist who uses a powerful Chinese medical acupressure that works wonders thanks to a powerful pressure!

For this type of patient, in particular for patients suffering from the muscular pain labeled as "fibromyalgia," I tried Happy Healing with success.

I then tried this method with patients who could take a harder pressure but whose condition was not significantly improved or improved without sustainability. Usually, Chinese acupressure can reduce pain and discomfort to zero or to 10 or 20% of the initial pain level. If the pain reduction is minimal, it means the manual therapy does not really work. I had the impression that sometimes, after the acupressure treatment, a cloud of negative emotional energy formed again.

Suddenly a magnetic, invisible "armor" of an emotional nature was set up again on the Body-in-pain, locking the muscles. All the benefits of the acupressure, all the muscular relaxation, and consequently the pain reduction, was lost with this terrible grip.

My initial reaction was to question the manual treatment I had been implementing. Perhaps had I treated the wrong points or zones with the wrong pressure?

After applying the Happy Healing protocol with success in these types of cases, I became more optimistic.

My interpretation was that emotions in the psychosomatic process are often a key factor, to a degree I could not previously imagine. Happy Healing was bringing the adequate solution: an emotional treatment for a physical pain.

Then, encouraged by these favorable results, I proposed to the patients who were in chronic pain, even if they accepted Chinese acupressure, even if the results were good, to try Happy Healing.

I asked them if they had the impression that their physical pain depended at least 30% on an emotional or psychological factor. When the answer was yes without hesitation, I knew that Happy Healing would be great for them.

I quickly identified three categories of patients for whom Happy Healing was not only a good solution, but "the" solution:

- "Untouchable" patients
- Patients who tolerated manual treatment, but without significant results
- "Over-emotional" patients or whose condition was linked to a strong emotional factor

These good results gave me great confidence in emotional healing. I was now beyond the experimental stage. The Happy Healing method was working well, and I had developed a detailed protocol.

I extended the application to three more categories. I proposed the method to patients who had tried other types of treatment without being healed. Happy Healing was in one way the last opportunity to improve their health.

I also recommended the method to patients who had good results with their treatments. The goal was to make sure that the psychic and emotional dimension of the psychosomatic process of a medical condition had been taken care of and not overlooked. Happy Healing was kind of an emotional health insurance which could be compared to an emotional detox: to cleanse all possible frustration here and there which could be removed. Better an emotional surgery on negative feelings than a real surgery on the body!

Then, I decided to propose the method to patients suffering not from a physical pain but from emotional and mental pain.

To be consistent with Happy Healing, the strategy was not to directly address the emotional problem or trauma, but to guide the patient in the body scan of phase A, to be aware of the parts of the body which were in pain or in discomfort under the influence of the emotional problem. Then the protocol was applied, with the naming of the Body-in-pain and the transformational phases.

As soon as the physical pain and discomfort was reduced because the frustration for the body had been reduced, the original emotional problem also started improving. I was using the psychosomatic connection both ways in a methodological go-between.

To treat the psyche, I was treating the body negatively influenced by the psyche. To treat the body, I was treating the negative feelings for the body. When these negative feelings were transformed, the body was improving. When the body was improving, the psyche was also improving.

I could now list six categories of patients for whom Happy Healing was very helpful.

Then, more and more, I used the method not only to facilitate pain relief on a physical level, but also to facilitate spiritual growth in connection with physical balance. I added three more categories to the six previous categories.

For patients interested by the spiritual path, the Happy Healing procedure was like a practical spiritual workshop. To modify the feelings towards the body, the method was assisting the patient to downsize the ego, and to put herself in the shoes of the suffering body, the Body-in-pain. As soon as the "I" of the patient was leaving his old perspective of "I, me and myself," observing the Body-in-pain, and understanding that the body was not an enemy but the instrument and the messenger of the cosmos, then, the negative feelings were released, sympathy and love could come in, and the body was rescued. Simple as it looks, this was the healing way of Happy Healing, a happy way for a happy goal.

In particular, Happy Healing in phase 5 proposes a channeling of the Higher Self which is delivering "Tips of the Cosmos." As you will learn in Part Two, if the patient has reached a high sympathy level for her body, she will receive these very valuable concrete instructions to apply in daily life. An impressive cosmic coaching which was also a spiritual blessing!

Then came the daily exercises. Once the physical situation had improved, the goal was to maintain this well being, this "better being."

The Happy Healing protocol was giving a very positive impulse. The happy self-healer could continue to practice this positive emotional and spiritual work by talking regularly to her body as soon as she received again some whispers of pain or of discomfort.

Happy Healing was teaching how heart opening could create a better emotional balance in everyday life. What a wonderful goal: not only for each patient but indirectly for the people living around them. An ambitious goal, which could help to make the world a better place.

With Happy Healing, it was possible to treat a patient in a holistic way, in a physical, energetic, mental, emotional and spiritual way, as was recommended in ancient medical systems, such as the Indian Ayurvedic medicine or the Traditional Chinese Medicine. Religions also lay emphasis on the importance of a sound spiritual practice, not only for the health of the soul, but also for the health of the body. Jesus was a spiritual teacher, but also a healer of soul and body.

Happy Healing is another wonderful demonstration of the mind-body-spirit connection.

"May all beings be free of suffering

May all beings be happy!"

— Discourse of the Buddha on Loving Kindness (Metta Sutta)

PART TWO

The Description Of The Method

"The zero pain option becomes luminous:
love more and suffer less,
love more your Body-in-pain and
the pain level will go down."

—Chapter 5, Guideline 4

"Love has not only an esthetic dimension,
a romantic or an ethical resonance…
It is a pragmatic force which achieves miracles.
Love is the great doer."

— Chapter 5, Guideline 12

The 12 Guidelines Of The Happy Healing Method

To better understand and capture the potential of the Happy Healing Method, I invite you now to discover 12 particular aspects, or guidelines, of the method. Happy Healing is like a jewel with many facets: let us see how Light can make all these facets shine and how all these guidelines can take you to a new perspective on emotional self-healing.

The 6 main themes of these guidelines are:

- Flexibility
- Faith-building
- Simplicity
- Dynamics
- Emotional health
- Spiritual health.

FLEXIBILITY

Guideline 1 - Session Format

At first, I was practicing Happy Healing in one-on-one sessions, lasting between 30 to 45 minutes each.

Then, during workshops on Chinese acupressure I was facilitating in Europe, I practiced the method in a group session. Each participant learned how to perform the body scan, to choose what I called the BOP #1. BOP represents the BO.dy P.art in pain. After identifying their BOP, the participants named him, then described him. I conducted the 6 phases of the transformation protocol without the need to know the nature of the BOP of the participants, except if they wanted me to know it. Like this, though the therapy was followed within a group, the medical information remained confidential.

I enjoy group sessions, which remind me of the prayer groups focused on healing such as they are formed in the Philippines in the "chapels" of the wonder healers practicing spiritual surgery.

I was so impressed by these breathtaking healing sessions that in 2009 I wrote a book about Filipino healers in French, *Prier Avec les Guérisseurs Philippins*, that is to say, *Praying with Filipino Healers*. My healing style and philosophy was quite influenced by these extraordinary practitioners. This paranormal form of healing that I witnessed and that I experienced with my own body was a precious milestone in my healing journey: what a spectacular proof of the Mind Body connection!

I remember that during the first workshop in Germany where I used Happy Healing, a patient who had still a back pain of grade 7 between 0 and 10 after acupressure treatment went down to zero pain phase after phase. She was completely pain free. Everybody was flabbergasted. So simple and so effective, and with the special bonus of feeling happy and full of love for her body and for everybody.

With this book, the method is now accessible individually in self-healing sessions: just follow the flow of the self-healing protocol.

Guideline 2 - Multi-Bopping

The method can be adjusted for any health issue. Any type of pain or discomfort can be analyzed, any type of negative feeling from frustration to anger and hatred can be detailed.

Then during the transformational process, feelings are modified, and even the appearance of the Body-in-pain as a person can change according to a subtle shape shifting. The personified body part, or BOP, can become younger or older, and his character or expression can be modified.

It is possible to repeat the protocol with as many BOPs as the patient is experiencing. Then the different BOPs can speak with each other in a surrealist conversation, which gives information about the patient's health.

It is also possible to repeat the protocol with the same BOP, but with another name and another description: the process will be different.

I use the expression MULTI-BOPPING to refer to all these application modalities of the method.

FAITH-BUILDING

Guideline 3 - The Carrot Reward

The patient following the protocol will soon realize how precise and immediate the consequences of her emotional attitude are, as if the cosmic power was practicing with the patient a "stick-and-carrot" policy.

If the patient is following the protocol, trying to experience as deep as she can the positive emotions suggested phase after phase, then she will be able to decrease the initial negative feelings towards her body, and from phase 3 to increase the positive feelings. She will see the results, grade by grade, tenth of a grade by tenth of a grade. Each positive progress in the feelings will bring a decrease of the pain or discomfort.

It is the proof that the Cosmos loves mankind: if we entertain positive emotions, we are rewarded! Love brings love.

These cosmic encouragements are not only pleasant to experience because the patient becomes more and more free of pain, but are also the demonstration that the method is working. The proof of the pudding is in eating it: here less frustration and some love will do wonders and generate the pain relief.

When the patient observes the first good results after phase 1 and 2, she becomes really excited to go further, and to enjoy new pain reductions.

This growing confidence, this faith-building phenomenon, contributes naturally to the self-healing process.

The zero pain option becomes luminous: love more and suffer less, love more your Body-in-pain and the pain level will go down.

Guideline 4 - The Beating Stick

On the opposite side, if the patient refuses to engage herself in this emotional work, or does it with a certain reluctance and resistance, then the method will not give the expected results.

If the patient does not want to be nice to BOP, the Body Part in pain, she will be beaten by the stick of Lady Pain. The pain will not decrease and could even increase if the patient's frustration are increasing.

Again, this is entirely the patient's choice. **"Love more and suffer less,"** but the reverse is true, **"Love less and suffer more."**

Originally, the patient perceives BOP as an enemy. The method consists in helping the patient to view BOP as good friend. If the patient continues to resent BOP as an enemy, the method cannot work.

SIMPLICITY

Guideline 5 - A Direct And Fast Method: The Magic Short Cut

The goal of Happy Healing is not to search to find out why the diseasing process occurred, why pain invited herself inside the body.

No psychoanalytic analysis, no exploration of past life's traumas, no link between a weakness in a specific part of the body and a corresponding psychic weakness.

Sometimes evidence will pop up, an explanation of the health issue will flash into the mind of the patient, and will reinforce the process of Happy Healing. However, it is not essential for the process.

The "magic short cut" of Happy Healing is more simple. Just concentrate on the heart opening taking place in each transformational phase, right hand on the heart. Just concentrate on this infusion of positive emotions. If the positive emotions are sincerely felt by the patient, then the Cosmos will respond, and the Body-in-pain, the messenger of the cosmos, will respond positively also: the pain level will decrease.

The patient will feel better and better, not only physically, but also emotionally. What a magic short cut!

Guideline 6 - Understanding The Misunderstandings

In life, understanding the misunderstandings often allows us to find a solution. Sticking to misunderstandings leads to blocks and dead ends.

The same remark is valid for Happy Healing.

Here the misunderstanding is to stick to the negative aspect of reality instead of also seeing the positive aspect, and of reinforcing the perception of it.

Pain can be viewed as a very unpleasant experience, but also as a positive warning signal.

Disease can be frightening, but in it is an adjustment process and a challenge which can make the patient stronger if the challenge is overcome.

The Body-in-pain can be resented as an enemy or greeted as a best friend.

BOP as a person with a name can be viewed at the beginning as hostile and not communicative. At the end of the process, the BOP can communicate as a warm and friendly speaking partner.

The healing process can look frozen at the beginning when negative feelings are culminating, and suddenly, when sympathy and love are building up, the healing forces may take a full swing and flush all the residual negativity.

This is why it is good for a patient who wishes to apply the Happy Healing method with the maximum chances of success to take some time to reframe her conception of the basic elements of the usual disease and healing scenarios.

DYNAMICS

Guideline 7 - A Slow Beginning: The Onion's Layers Model

Love is the ultimate healing force, but a force which is sometimes so difficult to trigger!

How is it possible to love oneself when pain is screaming inside the body? Anger, frustration, and panic are boiling...no room for love.

This is why to reach the blissful state of flowing love, Happy Healing is proposing a step-by-step approach.

Each step, each phase will facilitate slowly but surely the removal of all the emotional blocks and the creation of positive emotional inputs. At the end, love will be blooming and the solution will be given.

The process is like peeling off an onion, layer after layer. To get to the core, one has to be patient and methodic, and respect the layer structure of the onion.

Guideline 8 - A Quick Finish: The Swing Momentum Of The Healing Process

Though removing all the onion's layers needs time, acceleration can take place after phase 3.

The patient realizes in the middle of the transformational process that if there is "a bad guy," it is not the Body-in-pain, but herself. Huge discovery, huge flip-flop, huge emotional U-turn!

It is like an "Ego flush," like an emotional tsunami of repressed love which is freed when the emotional dam of self-protection of the Ego is broken. When the negative feelings reach their bottom usually at the end of phase 3, the positive feelings can build up more or less quickly.

If the patient experiences a rising sympathy for her body, it is quite good. If she suddenly experiences a jump of her positive feelings to 8 or 9 or 10 on a scale between 0 and 10, a jump to a high level of love for her body, then the healing process is in full swing and will be unleashed with a great momentum. Healing can be materialized instantly.

The process does not go forth as a lame wounded animal, as in the early phases. A beautiful bird flying again with full power is soaring into the sky!

EMOTIONAL HEALTH

Guideline 9 - Recycling Negative Feelings

The essence of Happy Healing is to convert negative feelings for the Body-in-pain into positive feelings. This emotional transformation is releasing the pain from the body.

We could say that the pain sensation is released, or the feeling of pain. The nature of pain is ambiguous: is is physical or is it emotional?

In the same way the temperature sensations are also perceived on two levels. A nice warm physical sensation, for example in sunbathing, can bring along a warm feeling of physical and emotional relaxation. Physical tension and emotional stress are diluted thanks to a pleasant exposure to the sun.

Empirically, we can verify that positive feelings for the body downplay the sensation of pain, pain, this very special emotion, the cry of the suffering body.

At first sight, the feeling modification should follow a linear transformation. Regression of the negative feelings, then progression of the positive feelings.

Experience shows, however, that sometimes it is easier to swing from one extreme to the other, from hatred to love, rather than from a little sympathy to a great love.

In this particular emotional alchemy, a high frustration may be converted into a deep love. This is the art of emotional energy's transmutation. The quantum of energy stays the same, but the polarity is inverted!

At the beginning of the process, a strong frustration, anger, fear or guilt may be identified – sometimes after some investigation, because the negative feelings could be carefully repressed by the unconscious mind.

One should not feel hopeless with such a discovery. It is the block favoring pain and disease. Now that it is identified, the Happy Healing protocol can be applied, and the conversion to a very positive love feeling could take place, unleashing then a strong healing process.

I have often seen patients after phase 3 overwhelmed by positive emotions, which might make them cry, once they realized the terrible misunderstanding which was opposing them to their Body-in-pain.

Happy Healing is a fascinating way to cleanse, to convert, and to recycle feelings and emotions observing the effect on the body through a self-talk with the body. The body becomes an emotional melting-pot and laboratory!

Guideline 10 - Creation Of A Better World

When the Happy Healing process releases pain efficiently for a patient or a group of patients, bringing physical and emotional well-being, it is not only good for the patients, but also for their relatives, friends, colleagues, and all the people they meet and interacting with.

One can observe a positive emotional ripple effect, the formation of a virtuous circle, of virtuous healing spirals. When one becomes free of pain, the whole community around the patient feels lighter and better off. Our emotional health affects not only us but also the different circles composing our environment.

Happy Healing works for you, but also for the people around you!

SPIRITUAL HEALTH

Guideline 11 - The Side Effect Of Spiritual Growth

What a beautiful emotional work, this infusion of splendid emotion-energies distilled by the Happy Healing protocol: kind empathy, acceptance and tolerance, compassion, gratitude, humility, joy, fusional love, liberation of all worries!

Phase after phase, the emotional cleansing work becomes also a spiritual work: less ego, positive feelings instead of negative ones, sense of connection with the cosmic oneness, increased capacity to listen to the inner voice, spiritual elevation.

This spiritual work as such is highly beneficial also on a physical plane. Spiritual cleansing and progression brings a peaceful state of mind, which lowers pain and unpleasant sensations, and which makes them tolerable when they cannot completely disappear, in case of an advanced disease, for example.

Even if the effects on the physical plane are not so noticeable, they are working at an unconscious level. Peace of the soul is a great softener of physical hardships. Spiritual achievements are, of course, a great benefit.

Guideline 12 - Love Is The Leader

Ancient medical systems, like those of the Indian and the Chinese, consider that the human being is made of several bodies: 3, 5, 7, or even more.

With a classification in 5 bodies, the first stage of a disease appears at the spiritual level, and then goes to the emotional and mental levels, and down to the energetic and physical levels.

Global, holistic health is a harmonious balance between soul and body health, and also energetic, emotional, and mental health.

Happy Healing enables this powerful connection and interaction between body, heart, mind and soul. Each time the Happy Healing protocol manages to release pain, it is the demonstration of the power of love on matter.

Love is not a luxury or a fancy emotion, a convenient illusion or a cheap feeling for soap opera. It is the real thing. Love is invisible… but its manifestation on the physical level, its capacity to restore the body, is manifold. It is a manifestation of the higher Spirits.

Love has not only an esthetic dimension, a romantic or an ethical resonance…It is a pragmatic force which achieves miracles. Love is the great doer.

CHAPTER 6

Happy Healing Visuals And Reporting Forms

To understand Happy Healing at one glance, take a look at the **graphic presentation** below.

This chart shows two curves: the pain curve, oriented downward, and the U-curve of the feelings for the body: first the frustration going down, and then the love curve going up.

The evolution of these two curves illustrates the evaluation process (phase A and B), and then the transformation process from phase 1 to 6.

Graphic Presentation

HAPPY HEALING - 8 MAGIC STEPS TO RELIEVE PHYSICAL PAIN & DISCOMFORT

EVALUATION

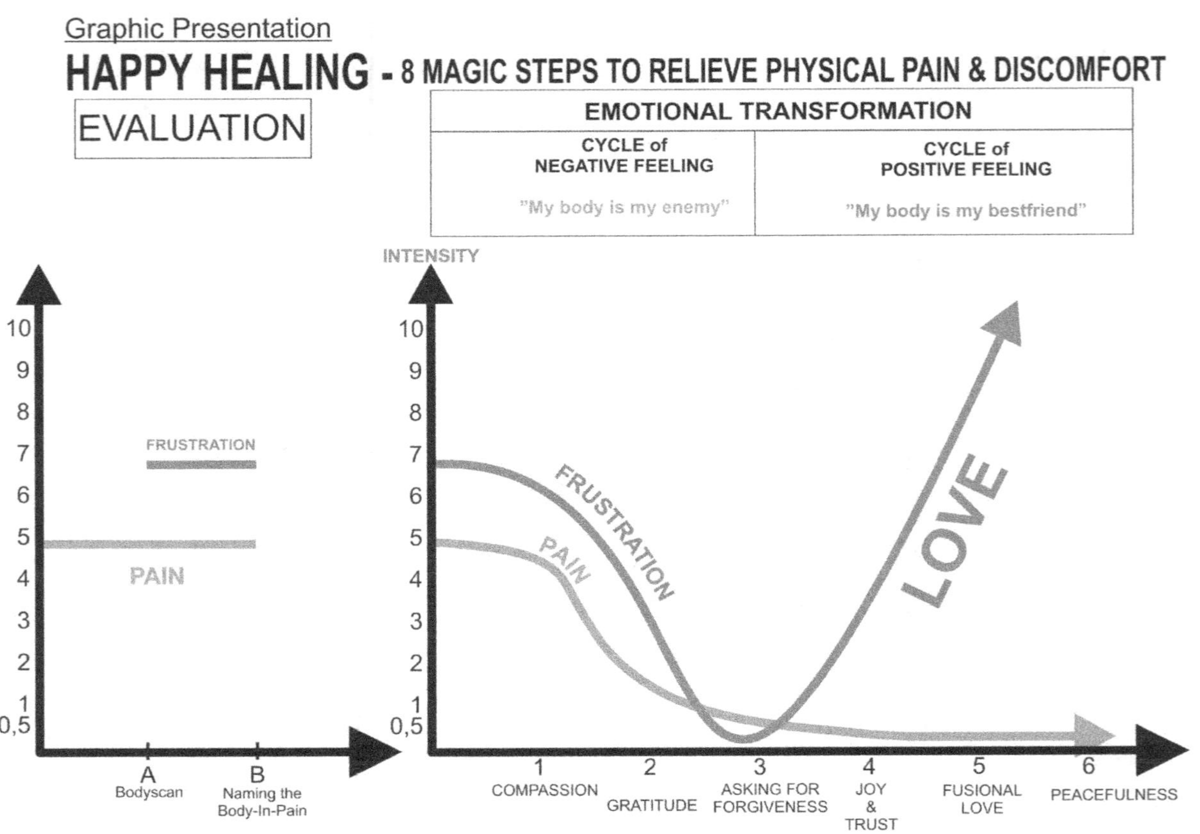

This is the great message of Happy Healing: pain goes down when frustration goes down, and when love rises.

There are two forms that help a patient to go through the process.

First, **the consultation form** with a representation of a human body (front, side and rear view) is used for the body scan procedure.

HAPPY HEALING
Consultation Form

Patient's name:_______________________________________

Date of birth   :___________________   Telephone :_______________

E-Mail   :___________________   Occupation :_______________

Session   :___________________   Date   :_______________

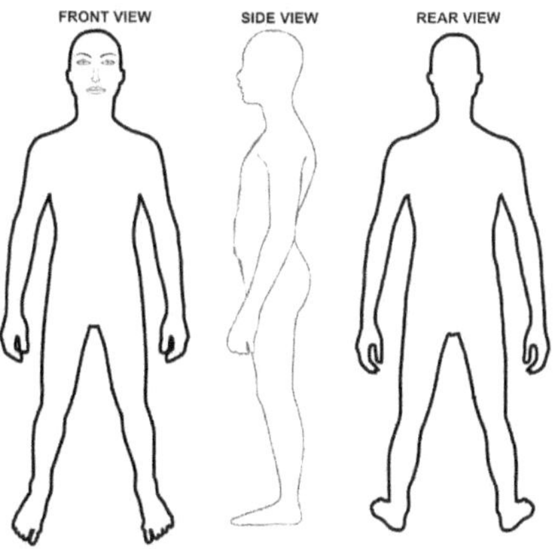

BOP's LOCATION (BOP = Body Part in Pain)
The body scan for pain and discomfort* spots and zones

BOP #1 is...

***DISCOMFORT CHECKLIST**

STAGNATION
Low energy, slow circulation, numbness, cold, blockage, restriction, muscular weakness, loss of control, feeling overwhelmed

BLOCKAGE WITH PRESSURE
heaviness, hardness, pressure, tension, STRESS
STOP AND GO
tickling, cramping, shaking, shivering, convulsion, pulsation, beats
RUSH
itching, burning, hot, radiation

* **The discomfort check list will be detailed in Chapter 10, which focuses on the body scan procedure**.

Then **the reporting form** is used for the patient to record **the evolution of the feelings for the body**, negative or positive, from phase B to phase 1, and from phase 1 to phase 6, **with, in parallel, the evolution of the pain/discomfort level** between 0 and 10.

An example is given in the Case Studies (Chapter 12, 1C). The consulting form and the reporting form filled during the session of a patient called Mary are both presented as an illustration of this transformational reporting.

HAPPY HEALING
REPORTING FORM
Phases A + B and phases 1 to 6

Name:

Date:

Session:

EVALUATION PHASES A and B

PHASE A. BODY SCAN
1. Identifying the #1 Body Part(**BOP**) in pain or discomfort
....
2. Grade on scale between 0 and 10 the **pain / discomfort level** ....

PHASE B. NAMING BOP and FRUSTRATION EVALUATION
1. Give a **name** to the Body-Part-in-pain BOP as a male/female person ....
....
2. Find out the age...............of BOP, and his/her **eyes**...................... and
   hair........................... **color**.
3. Grade between 0 and 10 your **level of frustration / guilt** ....
   towards....................(BOP's name)
4. Evaluate the **distance** between you and (BOP's name)...

TRANSFORMATION PHASES 1 to 6

	MENTAL IMAGE	EMOTION	HATE*	LOVE*	PAIN*
PHASE1	co-victim totally in the boiling pot	compassion			
PHASE2	cosmos's messenger physical sacrifice	admiration gratefulness			
PHASE3	double sacrifice, physical/moral	humility asking for forgiveness			
PHASE4	companion teamplayer	joy & trust			
PHASE5	higher Self's voice	fusional love			
PHASE6	cosmic oneness	peacefulness			

COMMENTS:

Hate* = negative feelings like frustration, anger, guilt, fear
Love* = positive feelings like sympathy and love
Pain* = pain or discomfort

Both forms can be used not only for a self-healing session, but also if someone wants to play the role of the **therapist** walking a patient through the healing process (a **professional therapist or an amateur therapist** wanting to help a relative or a friend).

CHAPTER 7

Overview Of The Method

Happy Healing is comparable to a surgical operation. It has effects on the physical body, but of a very special nature: an operation realized thanks to emotional tools, not the usual surgical instruments.

Evaluation Process: Phases A And B

Before the operation, you have the initial check up, or in more medical terms, the **anamnesis.**

Phase A is the body scan. The patient examines the location of all unpleasant physical sensations, painful or not, mapping all the BOdy Parts in pain or discomfort, denominated in short as "BOPs".

In phase B, the patient gives a name to the body part in pain (BOP) on which she wants to practice Happy Healing, the BOP #1. Then she evaluates her negative feelings for this particular BOP.

Transformation Process: Phases 1 To 6

This emotional operation of the body is performed by the positive emotions activated by the vision of the positive role played by the Body-in-pain.

The Happy Healing protocol proposes an articulate Mind Mood Management, a methodical chain of reaction of thoughts concerning the emotions and feelings for the body.

The mind management of the mental representations of the Body-in-pain's role enables the heart to feel positive emotions, which will transform the feelings for the Body-in-pain. Then the pain and discomfort relief will take place.

During the process, at the end of each transformational phase, the patient will be witnessing **a double miracle.**

The first miracle is the ability of appropriate visualizations to modify emotions, sometimes in a spectacular way.

The second correlated miracle is that each time a patient manages, phase after phase, to experience heart-felt positive emotions, negative feelings towards the body decrease and positive feelings increase. At the same time, the pain goes down, and the healing process gains momentum.

This is the Mind Mood Management MMM of Happy Healing.

Physical suffering becomes an option. The zero pain option is so simple: love more and suffer less. Love, instead of resent, your body, and the pain level will decrease.

Positive emotions towards BOP, the Body-part-in-pain

Here are the successive emotions activated towards BOP, phase after phase.

A. Awareness
B. Empathy
    1. Compassion
    2. Gratitude
    3. Humility
    4. Joy and trust
    5. Fusional love
    6. Peacefulness

Positive views of the role of BOP, the Body-part-in-pain.

Let us consider that the aching body part is the knee. Here is the thought and emotion process of the patient:

Evaluation

A.   My knee is aching.

B.   My knee is a person and a speaking partner. I call him Carlos. Carlos is hurting me and makes me suffer. Carlos has hurt my feelings, and I feel frustration. Carlos is my enemy.

Transformation

1.   Carlos, my knee, is a victim like me, and a victim who suffers more than me.

2.   Carlos, my knee, is the messenger of the Cosmos. He is sacrificing himself to give me the message, which is a warning signal. He is a hero!

3.   Carlos, my knee, is making, not only a physical sacrifice to warn me with the pain signal, but also an emotional one: I rejected him when ignoring his efforts.

4.   Carlos, my knee, is a cooperative team mate and team player. He is my best friend now.

5.   Carlos, my knee, is my guide and my mentor. He is transmitting the health tips of the cosmos to me.

6.   Carlos, my knee, is the Cosmos within me.

Positive emotional statements of Happy Healing based on the 8 positive emotions.

Here are the emotional statements made by the patient, expressing the new positive attitude towards BOP at the end of each phase. Those statements are enabled by the consideration of a specific role of BOP, which enables the patient to activate a specific emotion, which triggers the healing process.

A. Hello, my body, I listen to you, my suffering body, to all your pains and discomforts.

B. I feel that you are like a person and a family member and the name I give you is… I feel frustrated towards you because I am in pain, but I want to transform my negative feelings. I want to heal.

Phase 1. My heart is bleeding. I have only compassion and loving kindness for you.

Phase 2. Bravo! Thank you, thank you! Now I understand.

Phase 3. Sorry! Forgive me…I am completely changing my mind about you.

Phase 4. Together! We build our future together with joy!

Phase 5. I love you! What should I do concretely for both of us? You are my inspiration.

Phase 6. I feel so peaceful…I am liberated from all worries! I am one with the Cosmos. I am one with the divine presence.

Healing in Harmony

Those who know the Ho'o pono pono method of the Hawaiian Islands will recognize the similarities with Happy Healing. Ho'o pono pono is an emotional cleansing technique practiced in Polynesia in the Pacific Ocean, and in particular in the Hawaiian Islands. The goal of this mind body medicine is to facilitate harmony in the human relationships.

Such similarities exist because the two methods are likewise oriented towards reconciliation and forgiveness to overcome emotional antagonisms.

In Happy Healing, the focus is on the opposition between the "I" and a very special person: the suffering body.

The key words and mantra of the Ho'o pono pono are:

HELLO - SORRY - PLEASE FORGIVE ME – I LOVE YOU – THANK YOU

These key notions are also part of the Happy Healing protocol.

By following the 8 magic steps, by going through the 8 magic phases, you will cleanse your negative feelings and energize your body, emotionally and physically, with the healing force of love.

Enjoy Happy Healing, a happy way to reach the happy goal of self-healing!

CHAPTER 8

The Three Prayers-Meditations

Within this chapter, you will learn three prayers or meditations on the topic of healing and well being. These prayers-meditations help to understand different aspects of the Happy Healing method in a condensed format. Last but not least, they help to induce a calm meditative state.

Such a meditative state, which can be also called a daydreaming state or a light emotional healing trance state, is essential to hear this little inner voice, a manifestation of the Higher Self, which is the voice of the Body-in-pain speaking in the name of the Cosmos.

Many actions described in the protocol in Part Three are meaningful only if the patient is willing to access this meditative state. Heart opening, right hand on the heart, and healing mantras, astral clapping to thank the Cosmos, observing the attitude of (BOP's name), and possible shape shifting require one to enter and cultivate this meditative state. This meditative state, so nurtured by these positive emotions, will allow the positive blending of the unconscious and the conscious mind, and the healing process.

The emotional transformation of Happy Healing is surfing, so to speak, on the energy of this meditative state.

These three prayers are not part of the protocol, but experience shows that reciting them has many self-healing results. These prayers also induce positive emotions which can contribute to unleash the healing forces.

They can be recited or read as a reminder before going through the protocol. They will also help greatly to maintain the positive impulse of Happy Healing after going through the protocol.

Prayer 1. THE HEALING PRAYER TO DEAR BOP

This prayer is a summary of the 8 magic steps of Happy Healing. It is to be recited with the mention of the name of a specific BOP, the Body-part-in-pain, as a person named during phase B.

    A. My BOP (Body-part-in-pain), I am fully and carefully listening to the pain and discomfort which is disturbing you.

    B. (BOP's name), you are so intelligent and so sensitive, and you are so hard working for the family of our body…I respect you immensely as an exceptional partner.

    1. When pain or discomfort comes, you suffer so much, and much more than me! Right hand on my heart, I feel one with you, and I am all compassion for you.

    2. You accepted to suffer to give me a signal, a message from the cosmos. You suffer to tell me: slow down, take good care of yourself. I am so grateful to you for your sacrifice that you accepted for my own good to fulfill your cosmic mission.

    3. You accepted, not only a physical pain, but also an intense emotional pain, the pain of feeling ignored and sometimes rejected by me, because I was irritated or frustrated by the pain. Please accept my deepest apologies. I feel very sorry for my short sighted attitude. I understand fully now your double sacrifice and the greatness of your role. From now on, I will

make my best efforts to fully support you as you have supported me so well in the past.

4. Together, we make a fantastic team. Full of joy, we will build our successful future. You are my best friend, and we will do wonders side by side.

5. Please now tell me what I should do to change my daily routine starting today, reorganizing and simplifying my lifestyle? Which practical tips can you give me so that you and I have better health and a better life together?

6. You are my life guide and mentor. Help me to cross difficulties with courage and wisdom, and to rejoice and to celebrate in the happy moments. Thank you, thank you, my dear BOP. You are my life partner and my soul mate. You are protecting me with cosmic love and harmony. Thank you, DEAR (BOP's name)! I love you!

Prayer 2. THE LOVING RELAXATION OF THE TWELVE BOPS

Happy Healing proposes a new relationship to the body: a consciously positive emotional attitude toward the body considered in his material dimension, but also in his emotional if not spiritual dimension. This integration of the emotional intelligence of the body is the new portal into the healing process.

Here is a prayer for the relaxation of the body similar to what you would experience during a yoga session. In a yoga session, the focus is on physical relaxation as the yoga instructor is pointing out when doing a guided meditation for the yoga participants, "I relax my ankles, my ankles are relaxed." However, with Happy Healing, the emphasis is not only on physical relaxation, but also on loving the body, on experiencing a new happiness in the body.

Full of love, of loving kindness, as the Buddhists say, this prayer is addressing successively 12 parts of the body, 12 BOPs, which are perhaps not in pain, but which can relax and enjoy this demonstration of kindness.

This prayer is a form of self-talk with the body, with questions and answers.

Prayer 2. LOVING PRAYER TO THE BODY

My soles, I love you…you support my feet and my whole body, and you connect me to Mother Earth…would you accept to relax, to feel comfortable, to feel good? Thank you, I love you!

My ankles, I love you…you connect my feet and my legs… Would you accept to relax, to feel free, to feel good? Thank you, I love you!

My knees, I love you…you give flexibility to my legs…Would you accept to relax, to feel playful, to feel good? Thank you, I love you!

My hips, I love you…you connect my legs and my back right in the middle of my whole body, combining mobility and stability…Would you accept to relax, to enjoy your power, to feel good? Thank you, I love you!

My tailbone, I love you…you are the little tail at the lower end of my spine…Would you accept to relax, to feel free, to feel good? Thank you, I love you!

My wrists, I love you…you connect my hands and my arms… Would you accept to relax, to feel free, to feel good? Thank you, I love you!

My elbows, I love you…you give flexibility to my arms… Would you accept to relax, to feel playful, to feel good? Thank you, I love you!

My shoulders, I love you...you are the proud top of my back and the base of my arms...Would you accept to relax, to enjoy your power, to feel good? Thank you, I love you!

My spine, I love you...you are the powerful tree holding my body...Would you accept to relax, to enjoy your magnificence, to feel good? Thank you, I love you!

My neck, I love you...you are the precious little tree supporting my head...Would you accept to relax, to feel comfortable, to feel good? Thank you, I love you!

My jaws, I love you...you are the extension of my spine and such a precious instrument...Would you accept to relax, to feel loose, to feel good? Thank you, I love you!

My head, I love you...you are the crown set with so many jewels on the top of my body...Would you accept to relax, to feel comfortable, to feel good?

My whole body, I love you...you are the temple of my heart, of my mind, of my soul...Would you accept to relax, to feel like floating in the air, to feel so good? Thank you, I love you and I love all the BOPS and all the tiny little cells, which are part of you.

Prayer 3. HEALING PRAYER TO THE COSMOS

This last prayer is addressed directly to the Cosmos. In the Happy Healing method, the Body-in-pain is viewed as the messenger and the ambassador of the Cosmos, his representative.

I did not create this prayer, like Prayers 1 and 2, but adapted a prayer which I discovered in 2008 during a trip to the Philippines when I was asked to treat the Benedictine nuns of a monastery in Vigan for a few days.

Thanks to medical acupressure, I managed to relieve different pains and discomforts in the hands and arms, where the energy flow had been disturbed because of the strain of prayer postures held many times a day by the Catholic nuns.

The treatment sessions took place inside the community of the nuns, and before starting, we were reciting the Healing Prayer that I adapted, replacing "The Father" with "The Cosmos."

Here, the Cosmos is one general denomination to characterize the cosmic forces which seem to operate to organize and regulate the universe and life on earth. Depending on the beliefs and the inspiration of the reader, it is possible also to dedicate this prayer to the Father, to God, to the Universe, to the mysterious mechanism of return to good health.

This prayer contains many teachings similar to the teachings of Happy Healing.

The first teaching is that the cosmic power has the ability to create the body, to sustain life in the body, and therefore, is able also to recreate and restore the parts which are not working any longer. This potential reversibility of every disease is a great factor of hope. We have to ask the Cosmos and the healing forces to manifest themselves.

The second teaching makes the healing process seem more simple and therefore easier. After all, what is healing about?

On the physical level, it is an easy job, the job of a good plumber for living matter: cast out, mend, root out, open, rebuild, remove, cleanse.

On the energetic and emotional, healing is about the energy and the warmth of the cosmic healing love.

On the spiritual level, healing is brought by the power of the cosmic spirit.

The third teaching reminds us of a fundamental truth: the norm is not illness and pain, the norm is well being. There is an excellent reason for this: if we are sick, we cannot fill our mission on earth, which is to help others and to serve positively the cosmic powers.

Lastly, the fourth teaching is that we can introduce our healing request to the Cosmos through the intercession of BOP, the suffering messenger, our Body-in-pain, who is not our enemy, but our best friend.

HEALING PRAYER TO THE COSMOS

I call on you right now in a special way.

It is through your power that I was created.
Every breath I take, every morning I wake,
And every moment of every hour,
I live under your power.

Cosmic Father and Mother, I ask you now to touch me
with the same power.
For if you created me from nothing,
You can certainly recreate me.

Fill me with the healing power of your spirit.

Cast out anything that should not be in me.
Mend what is broken.
Root out any unproductive cells.
Open any blocked arteries or veins,
And rebuild any damaged areas.
Remove all inflammation and cleanse any infection.

Let the warmth of your healing love pass through
my body
To make new any unhealthy areas,
So that my body will function the way you created it
to function.

And Cosmic Father and Mother, restore me to full health
in mind and body
So that I may serve you the rest of my life.

 I ask this through my suffering BOP

AMEN!

CHAPTER 9

The Body Scan Procedure

This chapter teaches how to collect and analyze the body's unpleasant sensations in Phase A of the Happy Healing Protocol.

Sensation - the marker of any physical and psychosomatic disorder.

For every health issue, there is always a challenged somatic spot or zone. The body reacts. A physical sensation arises.

Investigating these sensations, these moving signals emitted by the Body-in-pain, can be compared to mushroom picking in the forest. One has to detect the mushrooms, see how they look, identify if they are edible or not, and analyze carefully each mushroom before picking it. In the same way, a patient must look for any sensation she can identify, and "pick" it carefully, take note of its shape, aroma, texture and scent as if it were a gift from Mother Earth.

This applies to physical health issues, but also to mental and emotional health. With a little training, a little curiosity, and a responsible listening attitude toward the messages of the body, every psychic patient can discover physical translations of her psychic uneasiness. Pain and discomfort are unpleasant, but they are also signals that there is a health problem on one or many levels: physical, energetic, emotional, mental, or spiritual. Pain communicates information about the whole body and person.

Sensations - the body's screams and whispers.

Such sensations are symptoms of a health issue. They also have an emotional resonance: they can be perceived as the screams and cries of the body, its sighs and whispers. Listen to the body as a person, as a sentient being who cannot talk with a human voice, but can scream or whisper with pain.

It might help to express the phonetics of the sensation in an attempt to capture the essence of a specific sensation. For example, to define an itching sensation, the sound "Scrtch, Scrtch, Scrtch…" can be articulated. By the way, this is how the word "scratch" was created, imitating phonetically the "scratching" sensation and movement.

Sentioms

All these sensations are living symptoms, not disincarnate clinical tests and parameters. This is why I call them "SENTIOMS," symptoms felt by the sentient patient, as first mentioned in chapter 2. The Sentioms-symptoms are the language spoken by this special sentient being, the human body, gifted with an emotional intelligence, when he wishes to manifest that he is in trouble. A SENTIOM is a sensation fully accepted, tasted, and honored as the "underground" voice of the body, of BOP.

This new consciousness of the Autonomic Nervous System through Sentioms helps the patient to change status. Instead of being a passive toy bullied by unpleasant sensations, the patient becomes an active observer of this global bunch of sentioms, composing a moving and complex coenesthesia variable as the streams of the ocean. The sentient-patient becomes an avid collector of sentioms, passionate about the cenesthetic masterpiece she is observing and subconsciously co-creating. The body is not perceived as a black box, but as an aquarium full of extraordinary moving creatures, the sentioms. These sentioms are messages to interpret.

Sensations - the Cosmos's messages

To give a broader meaning to this sensation and sentioms check up, the patient can collect all these multiple sensations not only as useful clinical signs, but also to assemble them as the messages of Father Cosmos.

These unpleasant sensations, including pain, are the warning signals that a change is to be performed to trigger the healing process. As shown in the transformative phase 2, BOP is the Cosmos's ambassador. Unpleasant sensations are the "bad news" of the embassy, the "good news" being that, with a change of emotional attitude, with positive emotions and feelings, the patient's good health will be back on track.

Six categories of body discomfort

As a practitioner of Asian manual therapies, and in particular of Chinese medical acupressure, I propose to group sensations of discomfort depending how the energy flow is affected within the body.

Six main categories: **stagnation, blockage and pressure, restriction, stop and go process, rush, and impression of loss of control.**

Stagnation

The patient can feel tired, exhausted, "down," with a **low energy** (for example under 4/10). **Hypotension,** stagnation, need to rest, difficulty to move, to think, to decide: a sense of **paralysis** which can be physical, mental or both.

She can feel a **stagnating sensation**, a "stasis" (for example **slow return circulation** in the legs veins). She can feel a retention sensation, an edema sensation (accumulation of stagnating liquid) in her BOP, impression which can be combined with a sensation of **cold**, in particular in the extremities (feet and hands).

The sensation of **numbness (no sensation)** can arise in particular in the extremities.

Blockage And Pressure

However, the pressure can build if the circulation, the flow, is blocked. Sensation of **blockage** and of **pressure,** also of **hard consistency**, of **heaviness**, and of **tension**, of expansion, of **swelling**, of tumor formation. **Hypertension** and not anymore hypotension. **Temperature** can increase.

Stress is a sensation which can be considered as the mother of all disturbing sensations: this feeling of stress and distress, of strain, of pressure, half physical, half emotional.

Restriction

The sensation of **restriction** applies when the flow is limited, though still going, and applies also to joints movements (rotation, stretching) which become **uneasy**, limited and painful.

Stop And Go

In this configuration, the energy flow manages to go through…and then is blocked again…until it is again moving forward, due to the strong pressure. This process of "stop and go," when repeated very quickly within a single second, may be denominated **"convulsions"** or **"shaking movement."**

It is a frequent case of energy disturbance, from **coughing, sneezing, shivering** with a sensation of cold or warmth during a fit of fever, **shaking** without control with Parkinson's disease. **Pulsations and beats** also belong in this category.

When the energy flow becomes weaker, no more "go" in the stop and go process. The "stop" position held for a certain time may be termed as "**cramp**."

The **tickling** reaction of the body can be considered the preliminary stage to a cramp and reveals an energy obstruction in the ticklish region. Though tickling is often associated with chuckles of laughter, this reaction is to be taken seriously as a warning symptom of an energy block already present. By the way, the process of laughing also belongs to the "shaking" family and finds its base in an abdominal "stop and go."

Rush

When the flow is too strong, too quick, the electric impulsions in the body are called **radiations**, and are usually painful (which is not the case of the opposite sensation, numbness), **warm, hot or burning…inflammation, itching** sensations. This the threatening quatuor: rubor, calor, tumor, dolor in Latin, translated as redness, warmth, swelling, and pain.

Loss Of Control

The energy flow seems impossible to control. The "command" does not function any more. The patient is depressed by a sensation of **loss of control.** She cannot "give orders" to her body, to her BOPS, as in the past. She cannot give the correct impulsion to her muscles and becomes **muscularly weak.** She cannot close certain sphincters or move her limbs; paralysis is not far.

This **muscular disorder** is sometimes associated with **tenderness** and an **intolerance to external pressure,** such as in massage, and in particular acupressure. This disorder sometimes induces an unbearable sensation of pain. In cases of "**fibromyalgia,**" it literally means "pain of the fibers and muscles." In this case, Happy Healing is very appropriate, as shown before, because physical therapies are not tolerated any longer by the patient. The logical interpretation is that the origin of the pain is more emotional than physical.[4]

Cancer patients

A pain-free cancer patient can qualify the abnormal state that she is experiencing with a specific discomfort: she often feels **overwhelmed,** invaded by an invisible and insidious conqueror. She feels hopeless, **threatened,** but she does not know how to react.

In that case, the sensation to be put in the "healing equation" is this feeling of being continuously overwhelmed, a physical sensation, but also an emotional one.

However, it is rare that even for an apparently "pain-free" cancer, no other disturbing sensations arise. Pain can be perceived and felt in neighboring body parts or BOPS. For example, a female patient with breast cancer will experience pain, or a burning sensation, in a lymph node under the armpit.

Mapping the body sensations with the body scan

The self-healing protocol explains how to report on a representation of the human body the body parts in pain or in discomfort, or BOPs and how to select the #1 BOP, the BOP to support in priority with Happy Healing.

It is always fascinating to see how easily patients without any particular medical training or background can give a quick and

---

[4]   Sarno, John E. *The Mindbody Prescription: Healing the Body, Healing the Pain.* New York, NY: Warner, 1998. Print.

precise account of the present "story" of their body in terms of sensations, the story that their body is experiencing, the narrative that the body wants to share.

To listen to their body, the patients are greatly helped if they follow the methodology of Happy Healing, with the right emotional attitude and focus.

They discover that they are their own #1 best expert on their sensations and symptoms and that they can easily interact with their body, thanks to the emotional transformation guided by Happy Healing.

What a great discovery! They can explore their whole body, and all the discomforts they are experiencing. They do not feel limited as in a medical practice where time is limited and where they have to focus on the biggest health issue, the most alarming symptom.

At last they have the possibility to listen to their body fully, carefully, and peacefully.

No hurry: just your body and you, together, oriented towards a Happy Healing.

Listing the BOPs

All BOPs are always willing to communicate…but it is the Ego of the patient who shuts himself down and does not pay attention. This is a great healing block.

Now, on the contrary, the "I" and the "Body-in-pain" are joining their efforts to find a harmonious solution for both of them.

If the patient is oriented in the right direction, with a few tools and hints, she can do wonders to take full responsibility for her whole health: physical, emotional, mental, and spiritual. This is the credo of Happy Healing: "I Heal, thanks to self-healing, I am in charge." A new philosophy of healthcare, inspiring, fun, easy, performing, and…free!

The patient is giving herself a treat, a grand tour of her body, this extraordinary inner estate, garden and home, that she usually has little time and, let us be frank, little interest in visiting thoroughly.

Now it is different: the time has come both to inspect the property and to enjoy a wonderful family gathering! Even if there is some anxiety: a few BOPS are not okay, and are manifesting in their corner…We have to see, we have to check…

So now the drawings are complete. One, two, sometimes six, seven BOPS are marked on the representation of a human body drawn by the patient on a piece of paper as explained in the phase A of the self-healing protocol. The record is a dozen BOPS!

An example of such drawings is given on the consultation form of the patient Mary in Cases Studies, Chapter 12, 1C.

Two types of indications are then written down for each BOP.

The first indication is the present value between 0 and 10 of this unpleasant sensation: 0, no sensation, 10, maximal intensity of the sensation. Important: this is the present value, here and now, not the intensity a few hours ago, or yesterday, though it is also interesting to note the different intensities depending on the circumstances.

The second indication is the date of appearance of the first symptom of discomfort, sometimes after an accident or an operation.

The #1 BOP

Once all the BOPs have been listed and documented briefly, the selection of the #1 BOP can take place.

The #1 BOP is the key BOP which needs to be helped first and for whom the patient will apply the self-healing protocol. Looking for this BOP of all the BOPs is a search for the healing Holy Grail!

The body is a superposition of different networks from the spiritual body down to the physical body…and the life energy flows through this incredibly sophisticated multi-network.

Now a serious issue: it is clear that the whole body is interconnected and interacting. Finding the magic spot which triggers the whole system at its best is amazing! Oh wonderful gateway, oh golden pass!

This is what all therapists are looking for, all acupuncturists are targeting with their needles: the best entry spot, which, after an appropriate needling, will restore the best health state in the energy vessels of the patient. Find the right button, press it, and the fortress's door will open itself…this is the fairy tale of magic healing!

For Happy Healing, this spot is the #1 BOP that the patient identifies by already channeling her Higher Self, a practice which will be developed at a deeper level in the transformational phase 5 dedicated to the Tips of the Cosmos.

The experience of an impressionist reverie

Let us indulge ourselves into an impressionist reverie.

We are immersed into a very particular sea: the sea of the unconscious impressions. So many waves and wavelets composing a mobile and fluid tapestry, a mystical music of the physiology of the body, unfolding into countless secret captivating melodies…a true Proustian experience. Explore your sensations freely and introspectively.

We stare at the hypnotizing aquarium of the deep psyche, but a psyche without boundary, engulfing the body, and the body's soul, all BOPs, intermingling body sensations, feelings, emotions and thoughts, swimming like exotic tropical fishes behind the glass windows of the Psychosomatic Grand Aquarium.

We are not any longer in the uniform material dimension, in the cold and mechanistic body machinery, even if it is an electrical or chemical wonder. No, we are in the realm of the subtle energy, the universe of the magnetic radiations, and we are now weightless, free from gravity, because we are floating like an energy cloud illuminated by the sun of the eternal vitality…floating we are, and our heart starts to beat: we are entering the land of emotions, ranging from the absolute stillness to the utmost excitement!

Yes, extraordinary impressions. Our body is existing on many levels, and we do not know how to grasp its true reality. Physical, energetic, or emotional? Or spiritual?

When pain is striking, is pounding, a feeling of hopelessness and rebellion may arise, with the crash of functionality of our body. This reaction is normal, legitimate, understandable. Time to move on now and to practice Happy Healing!

The Healing Equation Of The Evaluation Process

To prepare the transformational phases 1 to 6, it is quite important to examine carefully the data of the evaluation phases A and B.

The patient is carefully building up the **healing equation,** which will later allow the solution of the health issue and pain relief.

With a high level of pain and frustration for the body, the Happy Healing process is easy to perform. When the reality is more complex, as it will be looked at in the case studies of Chapter 12, a good preparation of the healing equation will be important to make Happy Healing fully work.

Three type of data to evaluate: the pain or discomfort (phase A), the description of the Body-in-pain as a person, BOP (phase B.a), and the negative feelings towards the Body-in-pain (phase B.b).

Phase A

In Chapter 9, The Body Scan Procedure, the 6 types of physical discomfort were described in detail.

When the pain level is high, the procedure is fairly easy to achieve. However, when the discomforts are too complicated to describe and of low intensity (1or 2), the patient must tune in carefully with the discomfort, and be careful and mindful in her assessment.

The pain or discomfort level usually goes down quickly during phases 1 and 2. However, a further reduction is sometimes more difficult to obtain and the progress is made in tenths of a grade on a scale between 0 and 10: from 1 down to 0.8 or 0.7, from 0.5 to 0.3 then to 0.2 or 0.1.

It is fascinating to see how the patient is able to situate herself with precision in a sub-scale of tenths of a grade, not between 0 and 10, but between 0 and 1.

Phase B.a Naming and describing BOP

At the beginning of Phase B, BOP, the Body-in-pain, is named and described as a person. Is BOP real, the voice of the unconscious mind? Is BOP an imaginary being?

Empirically, this procedure allows a dialogue with a speaking partner.

Readiness to communicate of BOP

This dialogue is not simple at the beginning. The patient is angry or frustrated towards BOP…and the reverse is also true! BOP does not look in the direction of the patient, turns his back, and is sometimes quite far. This is what happens usually in Phase B.

Then, phase after phase, the relationship warms up: eye contact is possible in phase 1, shake hand in phase 2, and a hug becomes natural in phase 3.

The ice is "broken" and the cycle of positive feelings can start with phases 4 to 6.

The visualization and the characterization of BOP is of great help to perceive the initial antagonism between BOP and the patient, and also later on to perceive the evolution of the relationship, which allows the healing process.

Topology: Spatial relationship between BOP and the patient

It is also possible to study a specific topology relating the patient to BOP.

During phase B, BOP is on the other side, on the opposite side, considered as an enemy or an opponent facing the patient. This opposition facing each other is the relationship to observe when preparing the healing equation.

Let us see briefly what might happen afterwards during the healing transformation.

During phase 1, compassion re-unifies BOP and the patient on the same side: they are both victims, but the patient still feels superior to BOP, placed on a higher level. At least the antagonism is gone.

In phase 2, the patient experiences admiration and gratitude for BOP: both are now "equals", on the same level.

Phase 3 favors a huge emotional U-turn. The patient realizes that the troublemaker is not BOP, but herself! Full of humility, the patient looks up at BOP who is now in the upper and superior position.

Then, in phase 4 both are co-operating side by side.

In phase 5, they are merging out of fusional love.

In phase 6, no more distinction: only a feeling of cosmic oneness.

Emotional and age characterization

In phase B, the patient visualizes BOP's character, usually reflecting a negative attitude: angry, rebellious, protesting, and hostile. Such features disappear in the following transformational phases: BOP becomes a friend.

The patient is visualizing a shape shifting of BOP during the process. The initial appearance of BOP in phase B can change or shift phase after phase. The age of BOP may also change: from immaturity to maturity (young child to mature adult) or out of rejuvenation (from a tired old person to a younger and more dynamic person). The age modification is a good indicator of the way the healing process is taking place.

Phase B.b

Expressing and assessing the negative feelings towards BOP

The patient is confronted to a subtle homework. She is confronted to a problem of "**psychic algebra.**" How to express her feelings for BOP and to measure them?

Let us review the healing equation to solve.

First, the patient must express her feelings. Not easy: many patients say, "This is my body, my body is a thing not a being, and I have **no feelings** for a thing, therefore, no special feelings for my body." Naming BOP helps the transition from no feeling to a feeling experience.

Then the patient can formulate a polite and "emotionally correct" statement: "This is my body, and of course, I like my body because it is my body." **Feelings are neutral or positive.**

The following stage is a state of **mixed feelings**: the patient, on one hand, does not like her body, is a little angry or sad about him, but on the other hand, wants to support him and likes him.

Here the patient must concentrate on the **negative feelings**, which are the healing blocks, forget for a while the sympathy for her body, sympathy which will be quite helpful for the second part of the transformation process. This is the only moment to lay emphasis on the underlying negativity. Not to maximize it, but not to minimize it. To solve the problem, we must not dodge it, but express it frankly and honestly.

The patient must really face the problem caused by her health issue, and articulate her feelings in consequence. Many times, a patient suddenly says, "Yes, it is true, deep inside, I am very angry, or frustrated, or irritated." Such a statement comes only when the investigation is detailed enough.

It can happen that the patient experiences **not one but several negative feelings** at the same time. For example: antipathy level 3, anger level 5, sense of guilt level 6, and frustration level 7.

What to do? In such a case, the patient can choose the negative feeling with the highest level (frustration level 7). This high frustration is like an energy reservoir: by changing the polarity of this negative energy during the process, the patient will "liberate" more positive energy to nourish the healing forces.

Sense of GUILT

A particular case is when the patient is **not frustrated towards BOP, but towards herself.** This happens fairly often with a perfectionist or workaholic patient, who is pushing her body too much.

Such a patient knows already that she is the one to incriminate for her body's reaction. The feeling to be evaluated is then a sense of **guilt**, which is a frustration towards herself. Some quite successful people, top achievers, can belong to this category.

Now comes another difficulty to dissolve this impression of guiltiness. One patient discovered during a session that her perfectionism, consequence of her ambition to be a top achiever and performer, was a great component of her success. Should she become more relaxed and less of a perfectionist, she feared that her motivation, and consequently her success, would vanish. She felt guilty and proud of feeling guilty, because this guilt was indirectly the great motor of her life. However, because of the body issue she had, she did well with Happy Healing and worked on this sense of guilt. With emerging love for her body, she managed to take away the pain.

Expressing and assessing the positive feelings towards BOP

Usually, during the emotional U-turn of phase 3, the negative feelings disappear and the patient experiences sympathy for BOP between 0 and 4. "Sympathy" will refer to positive feelings evaluated between 0 and 4 and "love" will refer to positive feelings between 5 and 10.

If the swing during this emotional flip-flop is really powerful, the patient is "catapulted" into the love zone, at a high level: 8, 9 or 10. Then the healing process is unleashed for sure. The pain diminishes significantly and often vanishes away. Such a new emotional state is a very happy moment for the patient. It will also open the access to phase 4, the channeling of the Higher Self.

CHAPTER 11

The Tips Of The Cosmos

In phase 5, patients are guided to channel their Higher Self. The detailed phase 5 is presented in the self-healing protocol.

Usually patients receive similar messages of daily wisdom, the same Tips of the Cosmos, which can be classified in eight categories.

The four main categories of these precious archetypes are the following:

1. **Re-centering**

2. **Contact with Nature and physical exercises**

3. **Diet and sleep**

4. **Social and artistic activities.**

The Cosmos likes to repeat the same basic truths. How encouraging! The truth is simple, and if we stick to this basic truth, we feel so much better.

The way to receive these Tips of the Cosmos is described in phase 5 of the self-healing protocol.

The 8 Archetypes Of The Tips Of The Cosmos

Re-centering

The first two tips concern re-centering.

Tip 1: Take some time just for yourself

The patient needs more time for herself, more "intimate" and "private" time, just for herself. During the channeling, BOP may suggest that the patient keeps a minimum of 20 or 30 minutes every day just for herself, even with a busy family or professional life: especially with a busy life! The art of doing nothing…except being oneself fully. During this "sanctuarized" time, the patient can recharge her batteries, worn out by stress.

Different options are available: sitting meditation, lying down meditation, just relaxation without doing anything, perhaps listening to relaxing music.

This **Tip 1** is the one which comes up the most frequently. It corresponds to the need for the patient's soul to be able to immerse itself in a calm spiritual oasis, where the soul can enjoy its singularity and at the same time its connection to the Cosmos…a useful step before talking to the Body's soul, to BOP personified with a name given by the patient. Before activating the healing forces energy field, a sacred preparatory pause is needed to connect with the Higher Self.

Tip 2: Do less

Downsize the agenda. Do only important tasks, de-clutter, eliminate unnecessary activities, take less commitments, do not over-schedule yourself.

Contact with Nature and Physical Exercises

Tip 3: Reconnect with Nature

Patients living in an urban environment need to reconnect with their body and with Mother Nature. Do not lose contact with nature, wander through natural landscapes, enjoy the sun, the woods, the sea, the mountains, and breathe fresh air.

Tip 4: Keep doing some physical activity

BOP as messenger of the Cosmos is recommending simple physical activities, depending on the patient: walking, swimming, bicycle riding, or guided training: yoga, Tai Chi, Qi Gong, soft gymnastics.

Repetitive movements or activities creating physical excessive tensions should be avoided: carrying heavy bags in case of a painful shoulder, wearing high heels in case of back pain, long sessions in front of a computer or playing a music instrument with the wrong posture…Obvious? Yes, for one who wishes to see with his eyes and hear with his ears, who wishes to understand and make a change, and who has the desire and the energy to do so. This is the point: weakness is the main obstacle to react positively to the indications of the obvious. Only love for BOP can bring the energy which will terminate weakness!

Diet and Sleep

Tip 5: Eat better

BOP also gives diet tips: eat less (for people who are not underweight) and better, eat less meat, less dairy products, and more vegetables and fruits. Detox programs of the digestive system are also welcome.

Tip 6: Sleep more and better

In some cases, some more sleep, half an hour or one hour, is also suggested.

In case of an acute pain, simple recipe: "physical" tips (massage, exercise) and go to sleep to let the healing take place, if possible with an empty stomach.

Artistic and Social Activities

Tip 7: Cultivate an artistic activity

BOP, the body's soul, needs to be nourished…and recommends often that the patient expresses herself with an artistic activity: singing, alone or in a choir, drawing and painting, dancing, playing a music instrument, writing…everybody is an artist because everybody has a soul and a thirst for beauty: BOP knows it, and encourages an artistic activity for the benefit of the soul.

Tip 8: Meet people socially

For patients who are a little too introverted by nature, or who become too self centered under the influence of their professional activity or of a chronic disease, BOP may recommend to spent less time alone and to engage oneself in social activities.

For extraverted patients, on the contrary, the tip is usually to reduce their external activities if they are too numerous, as seen with Tip 2: Do less.

Wisdom is simple and basic

The list of tips is not very unique or revolutionary. What is fundamental is that these tips are not given by an external coach, but are whispered by the inner voice of the patient, this secret unconscious inner voice connected to the cosmic intelligence via BOP. These customized tips are composing a simple but powerful cosmic healing plan. The inspirational way through which the patient receives them changes completely how the message is meditated, integrated, and put into practice.

The more simple the truth is, the more complicated it is to practice in daily life!

When I am guiding a patient in a one-on-one session through phase 5, the channeling phase, I am secretly smiling. I know that though the scenario is apparently dramatic:

"And now, dear...(BOP's name), tell me what I should do to improve our destiny, yours and mine, with the help of the Cosmos...," BOP and the Cosmos will answer in a very matter-of-fact way, bringing up one or several of these 8 tips, with some specific features. So when the patient answers after some hesitation: "BOP is telling me that I must take half an hour for me every day," I cannot help smiling!

When I first started to format the Happy Healing protocol, I was expecting that patients would channel extraordinary and unique messages. Not so...the most frequent message was: "Take half an hour for you every day, just to do nothing except be fully present to yourself without having to worry about anything."

Why this simplicity? The more we try to be one again, the more the solution is simplicity. Do not forget: reaching phase 5 is realized by many patients, but not by all of them. As seen earlier, the rule is the rule of sympathy and love: if the patient has not yet experienced a high sympathy for BOP, some sort of love, then the gate of the castle remains closed, and the patient will not receive a clear channeling from the Cosmos. It means that love is the key to access Simplicity and Oneness.

The Happy Healing message is simple: if your BOP is sick or in pain, just say hello to him with all your heart. Do not wait to be in pain: say hello to him everyday if he is in good shape but giving some signals of uneasiness! He will remain fit longer if you care for him. Do a little more than to say hello: have a lifestyle which makes him happy! Apply the Tips of the Cosmos!

To be sure to comply with the right cosmic guidelines, at the end of the channeling, ask BOP if he would be happy that you talk with him from time to time, and if yes, when? The answer is always a yes.

Importance of talking with your BOP during the first three days

Why is it important to continue the dialogue during the next three days after a Happy Healing session?

During the session, the connection with BOP is established because of the active emotional transformation process. If this connection is not nurtured, it will vanish. So, please, in your own interest, and in BOP's interest, keep talking to BOP in particular in the next three days after the session. Learn to cultivate this self-talk practice, as a daily routine:

"Hello, my BOP, (BOP's name), how are you today? Are you okay? What can I do for you, that is to say, for both of us?"

It would be good also to review the way you apply – or you do not apply! – the Tips of the Cosmos which were given to you.

You have the possibility to start another self-healing session with the same BOP or with another one.

All occasions to practice this loving self-talk with your body are blessed cosmic opportunities.

Benefits of a positive self-talk with our body

We all have experience with self-talk. When we say to somebody, "You know, the other day, I was saying to myself that…" we are reporting a self-talk conversation.

Some people speak to themselves using their own name, in particular to get some encouragement.

Mary, for example, will say to herself, loud or silently, "C'mon, Mary, do it, you can do it, don't be afraid or shy!...well done, Mary, I'm proud of you!"

Talking positively with our body, with our Higher Self, as in phase 5, helps us avoid becoming the toy of negative voices, the voices of unhealthy addictions.

Healing keeps at bay these different addictions, and honors the vital flow, the sacred flow, which sustains life every second.

Thanks to this self-talk practice, at the heart of Happy Healing, we learn to engineer positive emotions which will cleanse and energize and heal our body.

CHAPTER 12

Case Studies And Your Own Health Issues

In this chapter, different cases of pain and discomfort relief depending on the intensity of the signal will be analyzed.

This review will complete the study of The Body Scan Procedure (Chapter 9), The Healing Equation of the Evaluation Process (Chapter 10), and The Tips of the Cosmos (Chapter 11) and will help you to "customize" the Happy Healing process, with the help of the reporting form, to treat your own case, your personal health issue, and to express it in the terms of the healing equation.

During this review, for clarification, the report on the reporting form will be presented for some cases.

With **a high signal of pain**, the Happy Healing process will be more spectacular, with an impressive drop of the pain level in two or three phases most of the time.

Less spectacular, but nonetheless quite important to treat, will be cases with only a **small signal of pain or discomfort**. This signal can be perceived, with an increased awareness, but is sometimes confused or ignored, which makes the evaluation more delicate.

Third category: when the body does not perceive any signal, any living symptom or "sentiom," though the patient has been informed of clinical symptoms. Then the strategy will consist in creating **a replacement signal.**

1.   High Signal Of Pain/ Discomfort

When the pain is sharp, the healing equation for the body scan is easy. Usually the negative feelings are also easy to express. The difficulty arises when the feelings are so negative that the patient refuses to go through the process.

A. Excessive negative feelings

The story of Vendula in Chapter 3 has shown that if the patient is not only deeply angry or frustrated towards the Body-in-pain but really hating the Body-in-pain as a person, then the patient feels blocked emotionally. She can understand intellectually that some sympathy would help to lower the pain, but emotionally, she is trapped in a dead end, and the solution she is choosing preferentially is the surgical operation.

This book should help patients suffering from a high negative feeling for their body to reconsider their emotional attitude in a healing perspective...and to think twice before opting for surgery!

B. Difficulty to visualize BOP due to interferences with a real person

Another difficulty arises when the patient identifies the suffering body part with a person or a situation which is very painful emotionally.

For example, a man experiencing a sharp pain in his shoulder was going through a traumatizing divorce. This patient had identified his shoulder with his future ex-wife. He could not create BOP as a person, because he was strongly visualizing his wife, which was putting him in great emotional distress, blocking possible pain relief.

These two examples show that the healing equation is sometimes not so easy to prepare. In both examples, the pain signal is strong, and easy too report. However, the negative feelings were so high that the process could not get started.

C. Middle pain and evolution of positive feelings up to level 4

Among many examples, let us review an easy case with a middle level pain.

The patient, Mary, is a 50 years old woman, experiencing a headache of level 4 between 0 and 10, who named her BOP Laura and described her as a 30 year old with blond hair with blue eyes. Towards Laura, the feeling was antipathy level 5 (one grade above the pain level of 4. Usually the negative feeling level is slightly above the pain/discomfort level).

HAPPY HEALING
Consultation Form

Patient's name: _MARY_

Date of birth : _50 years old_   Telephone : __________

E-Mail : __________   Occupation : __________

Session : __________   Date : __________

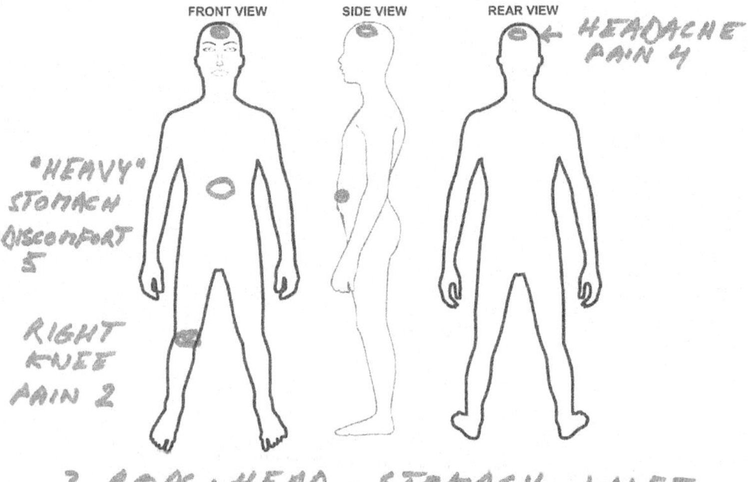

BOP's LOCATION (BOP = Body Part in Pain)
The body scan for pain and discomfort* spots and zones

BOP #1 is..... _HEAD_ ....

*DISCOMFORT CHECKLIST

STAGNATION
Low energy, slow circulation, numbness, cold, blockage, restriction, muscular weakness, loss of control, feeling „overwhelmed"

BLOCKAGE WITH PRESSURE
heaviness, hardness, pressure, tension, STRESS
STOP AND GO
tickling, cramp, shaking, shivering, convulsion, pulsation, beats
RUSH
itching, burning, hot, irradiations

HAPPY HEALING
REPORTING FORM
Phases A + B and phases 1 to 6

Name: *MARY*
Date: *50 years old*
Session:

EVALUATION PHASES A and B

PHASE A. BODY SCAN
1. Identifying the #1 Body Part(**BOP**) in pain or discomfort
   HEAD (HEADACHE)
2. Grade on scale between 0 and 10 the **pain / discomfort level** *4*

PHASE B. NAMING BOP and FRUSTRATION EVALUATION
1. Give a **name** to the Body-Part-in-pain BOP as a male/female person *LAURA*
2. Find out the age *30 y.o* of BOP, and his/her **eyes** *BLUE* and
   hair's *BLOND* color.
3. Grade between 0 and 10 your **level of frustration / guilt** *5*
   towards *LAURA* (BOP's name)

4. Evaluate the **distance** between you and (BOP's name) *Not in talking terms*

TRANSFORMATION PHASES 1 to 6

	MENTAL IMAGE	EMOTION	HATE*	LOVE*	PAIN*
PHASE1	co-victim totally in the boiling pot	compassion	3		2
PHASE2	cosmos's messenger physical sacrifice	admiration gratefulness	0	1	1
PHASE3	double sacrifice, physical/moral	humility asking for forgiveness		3	1
PHASE4	companion teamplayer	joy & Trust		3	0.8
PHASE5	higher Self's voice	fusional love		4	0.8
PHASE6	cosmic oneness	peacefulness			

COMMENTS:
Phase 2 : no more FRUSTRATION, some SYMPATHY (1)
Phase 4 : SYMPATHY INCREASES (4) BUT LOVE ZONE NOT REACHED → CHANNELING "The TIPS of the COSMOS" NOT so SUCCESSFUL
PAIN DIVIDED BY 4 : FROM 4 DOWN TO 0.8

Hate* = negative feelings like frustration, anger, guilt, fear
Love* = positive feelings like sympathy and love
Pain* = pain or discomfort

- During the process, the antipathy dropped from 5 to 3 and the pain from 4 to 2 in phase 1 (compassion).
- Then the antipathy dropped from 3 to 0 and some sympathy (level 1) was felt for Laura in phase 2 (gratitude). This emotional flip-flop from negative to positive feelings usually occurs during the next phase, the swing phase 3. The pain level went down from 2 to 1.
- In phase 3 (humility), the sympathy went up from 1 to 3, and the pain remained at level 1.
- In phase 4 (joy and trust), the sympathy remained at 3, and the pain was lowered from 1 to 0.8.
- In phase 5 (channeling the Higher Self), the sympathy went up from 3 to 4, but the pain remained at 0.8.

Here we see that the patient, Mary, managed to relieve her pain, but not under 0.8. What is fascinating is the precision of the notation: twice 0.8. Not 0.9 or 0.6, but 0.8.

Because the sympathy for Laura was not higher than 4, the pain was not completely released, which happens often when the sympathy is above level 5 and can be called love. For the same reason, the channeling of the Higher Self was not very successful: the "inner voice" is heard when the patient is clearly in the love zone (level 8 and above).

However, the fact that the patient had managed to be in the sympathy zone significantly reduced the headache from the original level of 4 to 0.8.

Congratulations!

D. Middle pain and evolution of the positive feelings to 10

The body part in pain of a female patient was a line on the whole back left side of the body from head to foot. The pain level was 4, like in the previous example. Her BOP was named Asha, 45 years old, blond with hazel eyes. The negative feeling was frustration level 9 (a much higher level than the pain level).

The frustration went down to 0 in the phase 3 as usual, and then the positive feeling made a big jump from 0 to 9 at the end of the same phase 3: a very powerful emotional transition!

However, the pain, originally level 4, was still high, level 2, in phase 4.

Because the patient was experiencing a great love for her body (level 9), she was able to do an excellent channeling in phase 5. The Tips of the Cosmos which were channeled were:

1.   Learn to say no

2.   Keep more time for yourself, 8 hours a day 7 days a week (much more than the average half an hour mentioned in chapter Tips of the Cosmos)

3.   Talk everyday to Asha, your BOP, before going to sleep.

Simple as it is, this "healing plan", addressed core concerns of the patient. She was an artist who needed to take plenty of time to practice her art, though involved also in a busy family life. This decision of being more assertive in order to fulfil her mission as an artist was like a huge emotional liberation and the pain level 2 dropped to 0 in this phase 5. Thank you Cosmos, thank you Happy Healing!

E. Importance of talking with BOP during the next 3 days after a session

It is very important, especially during the first three days after the Happy Healing session, to keep talking with BOP in a friendly manner.

A male patient managed to reduce to zero a chronic back ache of level 5. However, four days later, he complained that the pain level had gone up to 3. I asked him if he had talked to his BOP.

He answered that he forgot. Then he told me his frustration had come back.

I suggested the he repeat the procedure, alone, which he did. In 10 minutes, he was glad to announce that the pain level was again at zero! What happened is that unconsciously he let negative feelings towards his back come back. The result was the return of the pain. After 10 minutes of Happy Healing, the feeling was positive again and the pain vanished. This happy self-talk with BOP is your best prescription, your best medicine on the long term.

F. Easy process with young patients

I am happy to mention that with teenagers, the results are obtained sometimes very fast. They might reach the love zone in phase 2, with a reduction of pain to zero also in phase 2.

An interpretation for this quick response is perhaps that they try the process with the same positive attitude as with an exciting video game which is fun (creating BOP, talking with him), and the stake of which is huge, the liberation of pain. Plus, the fact that the process is a happy process with positive emotions! So they play spontaneously with great motivation and self-confidence, and the Cosmos is happy to reward them very quickly!

2. Low Signal Of Discomfort

By definition, a low signal is less easy to detect as a high signal. To add some difficulty, the cases are sometimes fairly complex. Let us distinguish somatic, psychic and psychosomatic cases with no pain and only slight discomfort.

A. SOMATIC CASE

Somatic cases are the cases to be treated only at the physical level.

Unusual somatic case

Sometimes the unpleasant sensation of discomfort is not easy to grasp and to define. What type of stagnation? Numbness? Impression of cold? Heaviness? In such a case, it is always useful to read again the check list of discomforts in 6 categories (chapter 9).

Somatic case with an option between two BOPs

The choice of the #1 BOP, the body part to treat first, is sometimes not easy to make.

When a patient experiences a headache and at the same time a heavy digestion, which BOP to select? Since the headache may be induced by a bad digestion, it seems a good idea to treat first the stomach, and then, if the headache is still present, to work emotionally on the head. The patient will learn to develop a sixth sense, to channel the Higher Self and to identify the BOP #1 to be treated in priority.

B. PSYCHIC CASE

Psychic cases concern patients whose main issue seems mental. However, experience shows that psychic cases are very often also psychosomatic cases: the body suffers also.

Where? The patient has to look for the suffering body parts. There is a similarity with acupressure, when some points are painful only if they are pressed. Here, the patient has to focus on her body to find the painful discomforts.

The body never lies, and the body is always present, as the ultimate filter. Even in psychic cases, never forget the body and the signals he is trying to convey.

Once the patient has identified the #1 BOP, she can launch the Happy Healing process. It will probably alleviate the physical issue and improve the psychic issue.

The healing equation of a depression, for example, will show that the main symptom, or sentiom, is a feeling of no energy, on the physical and psychic level. This case will be treated later as a psychosomatic case.

Traditional Chinese Medicine has already identified the physical issues of the principal organs in connection with a specific negative emotion. As defined in the Chinese theory of the 5 elements, liver and anger, heart and lack of empathy, stomach and worry, lungs and sadness, kidneys/ urinary bladder and fear.[5] When the patient is suffering from a specific negative emotion, Traditional Chinese Medicine can already predict where BOPs are potentially located.

B. PSYCHOSOMATIC CASE

When the patient feels that her case is both physical and mental, one can label it a psychosomatic case.

a. No pain but low energy (physical and psychic)

A common low energy case can be summarized so: "I am pain free, but I have no energy, on the physical level and on the psychic level. I feel weak and I feel hopeless."

This state of low energy is frequent for many people. It can be generated by a specific disease or simply by an overload of work and not enough rest. What to do?

For the healing equation, it could be possible to choose as discomfort "physical weakness." More energy would mean less weakness.

Here the recommendation is not to choose an indicator on a scale from 10 to 0, as usual, but to choose an indicator going up from 0 to 10, for example energy 3 or 4 to energy 6 or 7. It is often possible to raise by 2 or 3 grades a given low energy level.

---

5   Kaptchuk, Ted J. *The Web That Has No Weaver: Understanding Chinese Medicine.* Chicago, Ill: Contemporary, 2000. Print.

The body part may be the whole body, or a part of the body particularly weak or tired.

The negative feeling can be identified as the sad feeling of being abandoned by the body, let down, left on the side…this feeling of betrayal can be combined with anger or resentment.

The healing equation can be summarized like this:

- Initial sensation: energy level…(going up, not down like a pain/discomfort)
- BOP as a person: same standard procedure (naming and describing)
- Initial negative feeling: frustration or sentiment of betrayal by the body

b. Pre-burn out

A case a little similar is the "pre-burn out": the patient has the impression that she cannot make it anymore, that she cannot go forward. She feels stuck as a stubborn donkey who refuses to move!

Let us take the example of this male shopkeeper who used to be a workaholic, and who now feels not as dynamic as in the past.

His feeling of being "stuck as a donkey" was defined with two components: blockage level 4 on the physical level, and level 7, much higher, on the psychic level. The psychic spring was broken. The patient felt the need to refer to one discomfort not only on a specific level, but on two levels at the same time, with a psychosomatic coordination or correlation between the two levels.

The name of BOP, the whole body, was Didoo. No sense of guilt, but a great frustration level 7 of not being able to get things done as before. In phase 3, as often, the frustration went to zero and the patient felt suddenly a big love, level 7, for Didoo. The double feeling of being unable to go forward on a physical and psychic level went also to zero! The patient was relieved and experienced a great emotional release. He felt dynamic again.

The patient reached level 10 on the love scale in phase 4. He was ready for a great channeling in phase 5.

The Tips of the Cosmos were the following:

1. When coming home after work, take a shower, lie down and take some rest

2. Why not enjoy a glass of wine

3. Take the guitar and sing a few songs

4. Telephone a good friend

5. Try not to go to sleep too late

6. As always: keep in contact with Didoo, talk with him regularly

This healing plan was channeled fluently and received with great joy by the patient, who took a fresh start in his life and his business after a 40 minutes process "on the flying carpet" with Happy Healing. Really worth trying!

c. No pain but disturbed behavioral patterns like eating disorders

To treat an eating disorder, how to prepare the healing equation? Let us take a view on the two opposite disorders: anorexia and bulimia.

Anorexia and loss of appetite

First question: what is the body part in discomfort? For many patients suffering from this disorder, it might be the stomach experiencing discomfort - a sensation of stagnation, blockage, contraction, or shrinking.

On a psychic level, no interest for food and eating, and perhaps some form of dislike. This lack of interest in food can be also accompanied by a sensation of low energy and a lack of vital desires. BOP could be here the whole body, not only the stomach.

Then a BOP can be named and described.

The types of negative feeling for the stomach could be: frustration for feeling abnormal, fear of losing weight, of developing a disease, fear of becoming a misfit because unable to enjoy meals with family members, friends, or colleagues.

Bulimia and excessive appetite

This eating disorder is the opposite disorder: overeating, opposed to no or little eating.

The loss of appetite is often a permanent state. On the contrary, overeating and binge eating are sometimes performed in mini uncontrollable crisis during which the patient rushes on food, as if she could not help it. Let us work out the healing equation.

The body part could be the stomach which feels "excited" by the idea of eating, or the throat, or the mouth, which is excited by the perspective of chewing the food. It depends on each individual case.

The discomfort could be this uncontrollable "eating excitement" taking control of the digestive organs, and perhaps of the whole body.

The negative feeling could be frustration and fear of being submitted to an uncontrollable force, knowing the negative side effects of overeating: addiction, unbalanced metabolism, weight gain, medical issues.

During the process, the patient will sometimes channel direct messages from BOP, from the stomach, in case of a loss of appetite: "Do me a favor, relax! You are over stressed, and I, your stomach, cannot do the job you are expecting of me." Then, if the love zone is reached, a healing plan with the Tips of the Cosmos will be channeled, and a recovery process can start.

3. No Signal Of Pain/Discomfort And Creation Of A Replacement Psychosomatic Signal

In some cases, the patient experiences no pain or discomfort at all, but is informed by a medical doctor or a laboratory that some medical tests or radiographies are pointing out a health issue.

The patient is affected by this information not confirmed by an actual physical unpleasant sensation or sentiom. She can work out a "replacement" sensation in order to start the Happy Healing process.

Let us see what to do in two cases.

A. Blood in urine

A test indicates the presence of blood in urine (microhematuria), but the patient, a 60 years old male, experiences no specific pain or discomfort.

The healing equation is in this case:

- BOP: the body from the bladder to kidneys
- Since no unpleasant sensation is experienced, a replacement psychosomatic sensation is defined: fear of a growing health issue (bladder inflammation? bladder cancer? kidney issue?) Here, the initial fear is level 6
- BOP is named: Carmen, a 25 years old young woman, red haired, blue green eyes, tall, a little "power woman."
- The negative feeling for Carmen/ bladder: frustration level 8

What happens during the process is that the patient observes a shape shifting of Carmen, which shows how the healing forces come into play.

In phase 1, Carmen becomes younger by 3 years, and looks calmer and less "pushy"

In phase 2, Carmen is now 17 years old

In phase 3, Carmen is 12 years old, and seems a model of purity: a white angel.

In this phase 3, the patient feels a love of level 10, and his anxiety for a possible disease is no longer 6, but 0.5. The patient feels serene and peaceful.

In phase 5, he obtains the following Tips of the Cosmos:

1. Drink 3 liters a day and always carry a bottle of water

2. Practice yoga postures, in particular "the candle", feet up, which will improve the blood circulation in the waist region

3. Read on spiritual "pure" themes, entertain elevated thoughts

4. Keep talking with Carmen every day to check how the healing plan is applied.

This session will not solve this urological disorder right away. However, it achieves two results: the patient is more serene, and thanks to the "cosmic coaching" of phase 5. He will start to apply tips which will help him heal. Besides, his healing motivation is reinforced.

When the patient can « see » and « feel » the Body Part-Person as a separate and independent entity, with an autonomous life, possibly shape shifting, then she can heal this BOP so "externalized" as a healer would heal a patient.

B. Reduction of cancer tumor

Let us take the example of a female patient, 50 years old, who is treated for a brain tumor. She experiences no pain. She could work on the unpleasant side effects of the cancer, but she prefers to work specifically on the brain tumor.

Here is the healing equation:

*   BOP: brain tumor on the right side of the head visualized as a small ball

- Replacement psychosomatic sensation: feeling overwhelmed and stressed within the ball-tumor
- Feeling for BOP: here the patient who was a multi-tasking power woman feels responsible for "her" cancer because of her demanding lifestyle and career. The negative feeling identified is guilt.
- During the process, the patient visualized simultaneously a shape shifting of the BOP-person she named, and at each phase, a small reduction of the tumor visualized as a ball.
- At the end, the feeling of guilt was gone, she felt love for her brain, and she visualized the complete dissolution of the ball-tumor. She obtained also a cosmic healing plan, requesting to do less, and to take more time for herself as often mentioned in this cosmic coaching.

Create your own case study

Happy Healing is a multi-faceted self-healing method useful for physical and also emotional and mental health issues.

It is your turn now to build your own healing scenario. Have fun in composing your healing equation as a physical and psychological quiz. Then experience the emotional transformation of your feelings for BOP, and enjoy the new well being which you deserve!

CHAPTER 13

Happy Centering

I would like now to share with you the "Happy Centering" technique, very useful to "enter" the body energetically and to commune with him. It starts with the test of the energy Center of Gravity.

Strictly speaking, it is not part of the Happy Healing method, but it is an excellent preparation and complement to the self-healing protocol.

Test Of The Energy Center Of Gravity

I developed this test to help participants in my workshops of medical acupressure to develop their whole body perception. Then I used this test to help my patients to "feel their body" in a more "real" way.

It starts with the question which leaves everybody puzzled: "WHERE ARE YOU NOW?"

After a while, I repeat the question with a smile:

"Where are you now? If all your body was only one point, one spot, where would it be in your body? In other terms, where is your energy center of gravity, the place where you feel centered in your body?"

Lateral perception

"To help you to locate your center of gravity in 3D, I will help you, dimension after dimension. First, I will ask you to situate yourself by reference to a central vertical line. Do you feel centered, or slightly to the right, or to the left? By how many fingers or hand's widths?"

Usually three quarters of an audience are able to position themselves, and very few feel exactly centered. Most people feel at least one or two fingers too much to the right or to the left.

This information is then related to their health issue.

Vertical perception

I move now to the vertical dimension.

"Do you feel that your center of gravity is too much upward or on the contrary too much downward? Too high, or too low? How many fingers or hands?"

A perception too much upward may mean a lack of grounding, of anchorage, in link with an emotional off centering.

Forward/Backward perception

Then comes the last of the three dimensions:

"Do you feel that your center of gravity is too much forward, or on the contrary, to much backward? How many fingers or hands?"

The patient has now defined in 3D the position of her energy center of gravity. The way she sits, stands or walks, and her specific medical condition will be analyzed accordingly.

Ideal center of gravity

With this fourth question, the patient is asked to show where she would like to be. What would be the place of her ideal center of gravity?

This question is to be made when the patient has positioned her actual center of gravity and is now familiar with this spatial sensation.

Usually patients indicate the lower abdomen.

This empirical spontaneous impression is in line with Asian wisdom, culture, and religious and therapeutic practice: the energy center of the whole body is in the **Hara** (the Japanese term), also called lower **Dantian or Tantien** (the Chinese term) or the second **Chakra Svadhisthana** situated approximately two finger-widths under the belly navel.

It is possible to recapitulate where the patient feels now in 3 dimensions, and where she would like to be. This difference is the gap to reduce to feel fully balanced again, whole and one, centered within the aura, within a geometrically regular auric egg.

Oneness or fragmentation

The investigation gets further.

"Do you feel that you are one? Or perhaps that your energy body is divided into two, three or more parts? According to which type of fault lines? Vertical? Horizontal? Transversal?"

Sometimes, the patient feels that she has two or more centers of gravity, in particular, when she feels that the initial center of gravity is too high or too low. In that case, two centers of gravity co-exist: one for the upper part, one for the lower part.

This sensation can vary. The patient feels usually "too high," centered in the chest or in the throat, rather than in the lower abdomen. When she feels more at ease, more relaxed, more "centered" precisely, the energy center of gravity moves down.

Her center goes up, "pops up" when stressed again.

With the perception of two centers of gravity, it is likely also that the patient perceives an energetic fault line between the two centers. The course of such a fault line can be more or less clear, or more or less blurred. In case of back issues like a complicated scoliosis, the patient might perceive not only one, but two or three fault lines dividing her energetic, or etheric, body.

Whole body perception

After the test, the patient is familiar with, so to speak, her "auric skeleton," the structure of her aura, the energy body around the physical body. Is she centered? Off centered, and how in 3D? Is she one, or fragmented, with the existence of fault lines in her aura?

All these indications make apparent how the patient feels comfortable "in her shoes" or "in her skin," two colloquial expressions which refer to a state of energetic well being. "To be well in her shoes" refers more to the centering impression, and "to be well in her skin" refers more to the oneness and quality of the aura surrounding the body.

To be comfortable in our shoes, in our skin, to be present here and now in our body, well centered in the Hara or Dantien, to feel one and whole, all these sensory expressions are designating a state of excellent health, the goal of Happy Centering and of Happy Healing.

This energy center of gravity test takes 5 minutes to do. You can try to do it by answering the questions of the above questionnaire. This test is not necessary to apply the self-healing protocol. However, it offers many benefits. Here are four good reasons to perform it before a Happy Healing session:

Sensory training

Happy Healing is a method which evaluates unpleasant sensations in the body, and the feelings towards the Body-in-pain. Then the process is to convert negative feelings into positive ones, step-by-step, each time evaluating the evolution of the initial unpleasant sensation. The energy center test is a training to feel the body in its entirety, which constitutes an excellent sensory work and training for the self-healing process.

Many sensory exercises are possible, like the Buddhist awareness of the breath practiced in sitting meditation, but also the awareness of the heart beats felt in different pulsating locations, like the wrist, but also the temples or the ears, among other spots.

With this focus on the energy center of gravity, a true energetic acumen will be developed. This "cenesthetic" new sense, new ability, will contribute to the success of the self-healing protocol.

Medical information

Measuring how the body feels off center and possibly divided by fault lines provides useful information to understand the medical condition of the patient.

Happy Centering

The patient is motivated to improve the quality of her centering after taking the test.

Identifying the problem, a deviated centering, is important to find a solution, which is to achieve more balance and grounding in the lower abdomen.

Normally and logically, after a successful self-healing session, the patient should feel more centered. This progress can be measured quite precisely in terms of finger-widths or hand-widths.

It is a good motivation also for the patient to practice different exercises created in Asia and practiced now worldwide, like yoga, Tai Chi, Qi Gong, sitting meditation, and martial arts, which all have in common a better centering combined with a mindful relaxation.

Being autonomous and in charge

Practicing Happy Centering along with Happy Healing is one more tool to feel autonomous and in charge in order to monitor and improve our own health. This is the self-healing philosophy that Happy Healing is happy to promote.

What place do we call home, sweet home, in our body? How can we reach this wonderful centering, grounding and oneness within our lower abdomen, this magic spot which helps to generate well being and sound health? Happy Centering and the test of the energy center of gravity will help us to "come home" in our body, along with the self-healing protocol.

PART THREE

Application Of The Method

*"I feel ONE with the FLOW and
the ENERGY of the ONE"*

— Chapter 15, The Happy Healing Protocol

*"May all the Bodies-in-pain be happy again.
Happy Healing, dear reader, Happy Healing to you!"*

— Chapter 16, Recommendations After a Self-healing Session

CHAPTER 14

Preparation For A Self-Healing Session

BEFORE starting a self-healing session:

- **Sit comfortably in front of a table,** and prepare a ball pen with red ink and another one with blue or black ink, and at least three sheets of paper, to draw two representations of the human body and to report the step by step results during this session with yourself.

- You can also use the ready-made Happy Healing consultation form and the reporting form provided in Chapter 6 of the book.

- IMPORTANT: **Be sure that you will not be disturbed during about 45 minutes,** the average duration of a self-healing session.

- **This calm and concentration is essential to reach the meditative state** which will help you to achieve the emotional transformation, as if you were "on a flying carpet." For the first session, you need more time since you are discovering the method.

- It is also important to **write down what happens during the process** on the reporting form (the one which is provided or the one you create). This track record helps you to ground the process. After the session, it will be a good reminder of what happened, what you discovered about your health, and about your self-healing capacity.

- **Feel happy to soon be relieved from pain and discomfort!**

DURING THE SESSION

- Go through the EVALUATION (phase A and phase B), then through phases 1 and 2 of the TRANSFORMATION.
- If you feel comfortable with the method, go further. If your positive feelings are increasing, you can go through phase 6.
- Trust the technique, which has helped hundreds of patients. The three ingredients to bring from your side are: **focus, positivity, and the wish to heal.**
- Just get on board and **have fun** during this emotional trip!
- To achieve the **emotional healing transformation**, phase after phase, a **basic pattern** will be used combining **visualizations, emotional experiences, and mindful observations.**

The sequence:

- **Statement**
  - The visualization of the role of the Body-in-pain

- **Heart Opening**
  - The positive emotional transformation

- **Healing Mantra**
  - The healing sentence I am pronouncing silently or loudly

- **Body Magnetization** (phases 4 to 6)
  - Magnetization with the left hand above the physical BOP

- **Feelings and Pain Evaluation**
  - The results at the end of each phase: better feelings and pain reduction

- **Astral Clapping**
  - Thanking the cosmos for the good results obtained

- **Talking Terms**
  - The possibility to talk with the Body-in-pain from being not on talking terms to hugging each other

- **Shape Shifting**
  - Modification of the appearance of the person behind the Body-in-pain, sentient being who received a name

- **Emotional Work Review**
  - Recapitulation of the emotional work achieved phase after phase

Through the 8 steps, the main actor of the self-healing protocol is "I". That is to say, YOU, represented at the first person "I".

"I" is thinking, feeling, doing, transforming. You are the subject of the protocol, the self-healing patient solving his/her health issues.

You are healing yourself: **you are the healer.**

Here are the orientations of your self-healing homework:

"I" am thinking and visualizing: **Statement, Emotional Work Review**

"I" am feeling and transforming: **Heart opening and Healing Mantra, Body Magnetization, Astral Clapping, Talking Terms**

"I" am feeling and observing: **Feeling and Pain Evaluation, Shape Shifting**

The Happy Healing protocol has already been introduced in Chapter 6 and Chapter 7.

Here a quick reminder of the 8 magic steps of Happy Healing:

Evaluation

Phase A. Body Scan and pain/discomfort evaluation

Phase B. Naming the Body-in-pain and evaluating the negative feelings/frustrations towards the body which have been generated because of the pain/ discomfort

Transformation

CYCLE OF NEGATIVE FEELING. PHASES 1 TO 3
Phase 1. Compassion
Phase 2. Gratitude
Phase 3. Humility and Asking for forgiveness

CYCLE OF POSITIVE FEELING. PHASES 4 TO 6
Phase 4. Joy and Trust
Phase 5. Fusional Love
Phase 6. Peacefulness and Liberation

Are you ready? Enter the first of the process, evaluation phase A, the body scan procedure.

HAPPY HEALING OUT OF YOUR PAIN, OUT OF YOUR DISCOMFORT!

As you begin to use Happy Healing, you may want to start by using the much shorter 4 step version of the protocol. It is a wonderful way to familiarize yourself with the protocol and your own healing.

Visit **www.HappyHealingBook.com/bonus** to receive your copy of this bonus mini-protocol.

CHAPTER 15

The Happy Healing Protocol

Evaluation Phases A And B

PHASE A. Body Scan and pain/discomfort evaluation

I enter a calm meditative state and I pay thorough attention to my body.

With this awareness, I honor my body, and I recognize his needs.

Drawing The Body With Mindfulness

On a first sheet of paper, I draw a simple representation of the front view of my body. Then on a second sheet, the rear view, the back view.

Doing so, I start consciously to scrutinize what is going on in my body. I am performing the body scan described in chapter 9.

I welcome a flow of various sensations. I greet them and observe them carefully, taking all the necessary time.

Spotting The Painful Zones

On the front and the rear view of the human body drawn by me, with a red ink ball pen, I mark all the points, zones, and lines which are in pain in my body. Alternatively, I can also use the drawings of the consultation form provided in Chapter 6 and in the appendix.

Large zone

Sometimes, the painful zone is a large one without clear boundaries, for example: left side of the body, or right side of the torso.

Twin body parts

A specific case is the case of twin and symmetrical parts of the body: feet, ankles, knees, hips, elbows, shoulders, and so on.

I evaluate if the pain or discomfort is identical in both twin parts. If so, I can refer to only one zone for the twin parts, for example "feet".

If my pain and sensation is different in each of the two body parts, I choose one body part with 2 sub-body parts, for example feet/right foot, left foot. I will give a different name to each of the two body parts.

I write down then **the level of pain experienced in each spot on a scale between 0 and 10.**

What counts is the message of the body in the present moment, not a few hours ago.

I mention briefly, if possible, when (how many hours, days, weeks, months, or years) the pain started. This exploration, in medical terms, is called an anamnesis: the track record of the painful spots.

By doing this body scan with full awareness, I realize that I am communicating better with the emotional intelligence of my body, because I am listening to all his messages of distress, that is to say the pain signals.

Observing the pain and the painful zone as an external observer is already a process which helps me to overcome the pain, not be the pain's puppet and toy.

Calming the mind allows me to calm my emotions and my feelings, including pain, this very special sensation/emotion.

Spotting The Discomfort Zones

Once all painful spots have been listed and evaluated, I repeat the same process with the discomfort zones. Physical discomforts are the non-painful, but unpleasant sensations experienced by the body. Pain, in itself a strong discomfort, has already been reported.

I use a pen of a different color to do this, and I evaluate **the intensity of the discomfort on a scale between 0 and 10.**

Here a short list of possible physical discomforts, which are detailed in chapter 10:

warmth or coldness, hardness or softness, heaviness or lack of consistency, itching, stagnation, lack of flow, numbness, weak energy, shaking or trembling sensation, or on the contrary irradiation, flushing or burning sensation.

I list also possible psychic discomforts concerning the body: sensation of being overwhelmed or out of control, sensation of disorder or of unbalance.

Identifying The Spot Number One

On the two drawings of my body, I observe all the painful and uncomfortable spots that I have been marking. Usually 2 or 3 spots, or more. Rarely no spot at all: the body has a lot to say through different signals, if we accept to listen to him and hear him.

I will now select the spot number one.

This is the priority spot which needs the most emotional help and support from me right now. It is also the magic spot which, if it feels better, will have the maximum positive impact on all other spots in pain or discomfort.

All these spots are also called "BOPs", BOP stands for "BO dy P art in pain or discomfort."

This priority spot, or **#1 BOP,** is usually the most painful spot, but not necessarily.

To identify this magic spot, the improvement of which will leverage best the well being of all the other BOPs of my body, I carefully review the main critical spots. Each time, I speak mentally to each one of them and listen to the answer that I might perceive in a sort of daydreaming mode.

I make my choice: my BOP number one on which I will work by priority is _____.

Emotional Work Review

This interest for my body, this respect of the signals emitted, this recognition of the suffering going on, the display of my loving kindness, is a blessing for my body.

My whole Body-in-pain feels happy because I take the time to listen to all the distress signals. He feels taken care of and protected.

Phase B. Naming Of Bop And Negative Feeling Evaluation After Naming Bop

To acknowledge the fact that I perceive the Body-in-pain as a sentient being, as a person, I will now give a name to #1 BOP. The name can be a male or a female name, a name frequently given or unusual in whatever language.

Twin body parts

If I decided to differentiate two twin body parts, for example right foot and left foot, I will choose a name for each BOP, which could be a name already used for twins, such as "Tom and Jerry". I will go through the protocol with these two mini BOPs.

Avoid Names Of Well Known Persons

I avoid giving BOP the name of my relatives, friends, partners, colleagues or pets.

If such a name comes to my mind, I will note it, but I will not choose it for the Happy Healing process. It is often the name of somebody with whom a psychic complication created a physical pain or discomfort, and I wish to avoid a possible transference of negativity to BOP.

Avoid Names With A Negative Meaning

I will not use familiar nicknames, names with repetition of the same syllable, or names too complicated, funny sounding, or out of use. Often, these types of names are expressing some form of negativity toward BOP. If it is clearly not kind, it translates the negative feeling I feel for BOP. Since I wish to transform this negative feeling, I look for a neutral name. I write it down when found, for example JIM or MARY.

I make a last check: is the name found not associated with somebody I know well?

Is it neutral? Does it sound positive?

It is important to find the right name, which will assist me in conducting the emotional transformation, with a precise healing effect. For this special subtle transformational work of Happy Healing, the vibration of the name should help and not weaken the healing forces.

Description Of The Body-In-Pain, Bop, As A Person

My BOP, my body-in-pain now has a name. I perceive him as a person.
I look at him carefully and I describe him:

AGE

BOP may be as old as me, but also very old, more than 100 years old, or very young, as a child or baby.

This age will probably change during the Happy Healing Process, and will show a healing evolution. I will note this « shape shifting » when it occurs.

HAIR and EYE COLOR

I observe the color of BOP's hair and eyes. I write this down. By doing so, I better visualize BOP. Therefore, it is easier for me to analyze my true feelings for him.

Double Perception Of Bop

I perceive now BOP in two dimensions.

The first BOP is the part of my Body-in-pain, my physical BOP.

The second BOP is the person BOP that I just created with a name. In one way, this is like "the spirit" or "the soul" of the physical BOP. BOP's soul is an image for the emotional intelligence of my body, so sensitive to the feelings I have for him.

This enlarged perception of BOP allows me to better separate myself, my « I », my « ego », from my Body-in-pain and simultaneously to better connect to him. I split myself in order to better re-unify myself.

Negative Feeling Evaluation

I observe now my feelings for my Body-in-pain as explained in the healing equation of chapter 10.

Perhaps I feel some **mixed feelings**: some sympathy ("this is my body after all"), but also some frustration ("my body is somehow betraying me and creating trouble").

The higher the pain, the higher the frustration.

The smaller the discomfort, the smaller the frustration.

This frustration can also be hatred, anger and resentment.

In some cases, I feel guilt toward my Body-in-pain, because I know I have pushed my body too much, beyond his normal capacity. Guilt is also a frustration, not directed toward the body, but toward myself.

In this phase, I try to evaluate my gut feeling, my real frustration for my body which is giving me pain and who does not serve me as usual.

I took for granted before that my body works for me in a smooth way, 24 hours a day, as a silent and efficient servant, as an obedient robot. And with the pain I realize that my body does not want to work so well as in the past! Somehow, I feel abandoned and perhaps betrayed.

I do not try to be polite, to be nice. It is not about trying to be "emotionally correct": I just express my irritation and my perception of being disturbed by my dysfunctioning body. I don't repress this frustration, which is normal, usual, and legitimate; I allow it to come out.

So, on a scale between 0 and 10, **my frustration for BOP is…**

Talking Terms

If I try to speak now to (BOP's name), it will be perhaps difficult. Perhaps BOP will be far away, or turning his back to me. BOP is retaliating against my negative attitude. I don't like him…and he doesn't like me, as simple as that. So we are not on talking terms at the beginning.

I experience frustration and (BOP's name) also experiences frustration toward me. BOP's attitude mirrors my attitude.

This is the therapeutic leverage of Happy Healing: by improving my emotional attitude toward BOP, BOP feels more positive toward me, and the healing can take place.

Emotional Work Review

I managed to connect with my body as a sentient being, and I named my BOP.

With equanimity, I watched the emotional reality as it is: the pain or discomfort triggered frustration and negative feelings towards my body.

I feel that it is an important block on the healing path. I will now engage myself into a six phase emotional transformation process to dissolve this block.

Transformation Phases 1 To 6

I will now do visualizations which will transform my emotional attitude towards my Body-in-pain. This is the Mind Mood Management MMM of the method Happy Healing, which has helped hundreds of patients to heal through these visualizations.

I will accept the different assumptions behind these visualizations without questioning them. The relevance of these assumptions will be clear to me when the pain starts to come down.

The proof of the pudding is in eating it, and the proof of Happy Healing is in feeling better emotionally and physically.

Cycle Of Negative Feelings Phases 1 To 3

For each transformational phase, the same sequence will be followed:
- Statement
- Heart opening
- Healing Mantra
- Body magnetization (phase 4 to 6)
- Feeling Evaluation
- Pain Evaluation
- Astral clapping
- Talking terms
- Shape shifting
- Emotional Work Review

Phase 1. Compassion

STATEMENT

"I realize that (BOP's name) is also a victim like me, a victim who suffers more than me."

Imagine a hot pan on a fire containing boiling water, a hot pan with a long handle.

BOP is completely immersed in the boiling water. I am only holding the extremity of the handle.

When the pain/discomfort is there, BOP is suffering and suffering much more than me because he is entirely in the boiling water, he is the whole painful spot. Myself, I am partially disturbed by the pain, but my situation is different. I can read, watch a film, or talk with friends to forget the pain. I am only holding the handle of the pan: a little warm, but bearable.

HEART OPENING

I now put my right hand on my heart.

HEALING MANTRA

"I am sending all my compassion to (BOP's name) who is a victim like me, a victim who suffers more than me."

I stay attuned in this powerful and warm emotional stream of compassion toward BOP. I stay attuned and wait until I feel that a deep compassion has been flowing from my heart to (BOP's name).

All my being enjoys this infusion of love and this warm emotional stream warming me up body and soul.

Then I do **two evaluations.**

FRUSTRATION

My frustration level which was…on a scale from 0 to 10 is lower and is now…

PAIN/ DISCOMFORT

My pain or discomfort level which was…is also lower and is now…

For example, if the pain level was originally 7 in phase A, and the frustration/strong antipathy also 7 in phase B, after the compassion phase 1, the frustration might go down to 5 and the pain also to 5.

This is the double miracle of "Happy Healing": negative and positive feelings can be modified through visualizations. This is the special Mind Mood Management MMM of Happy Healing.

Feelings less and **less negative** during phases 1 to 3 and more and **more positive** during phases 4 to 6 translate into a **reduction of pain and discomfort.**

These show the correlation miracle between feelings toward the body and unpleasant physical sensations in the body.

Pain seems to be both a special physical sensation and a specific emotion. An emotional improvement brings an improvement on the physical side.

The good news: positivity is the mother of positivity.

ASTRAL CLAPPING

To thank the healing forces of the Cosmos, which have manifested themselves by this improvement, **I gently clap my hands in gratitude** in a state of light emotional trance.

TALKING TERMS

The improvement obtained allows me to see a BOP closer and more friendly to me. I can now make **eye contact**, if not shake BOP's hand.

SHAPE SHIFTING

I observe possible changes: If BOP was very old, he will probably be younger now. If he was too young, lacking maturity, he will perhaps be older. His character might also be improved.

EMOTIONAL WORK REVIEW

I have made a great step forward with this first heart opening of the transformational phase 1.

I have been given a healing manifestation.

My positive emotions, compassion for phase 1, decreased my negative feeling for BOP and simultaneously my pain/discomfort level.

Thank you, Cosmos (or as appropriate for everyone: Thank you Universe, thank you God, thank you mysterious Mechanism of Return to Good Health…).

My confidence in self-healing is building up.

Phase 2. Gratitude

STATEMENT

"I realize that (BOP's name) is the messenger and the ambassador of the Cosmos. The message of this pain/discomfort signal is a wake up call. Something is wrong in my life, I must adjust.

(BOP's name) is only an instrument of the Cosmos and personally neither enjoys sending me pain nor enjoys experiencing pain.

I am so grateful to (BOP's name), a hero who has sacrificed himself physically to transmit to me the pain/discomfort signal sent by the Cosmos.

Thanks to this sacrifice, I feel now a connection with the Cosmos, which wants me to change something in my life to allow me to again be in good health.

I am twice grateful: to the messenger, (BOP's name), and to the Cosmos, which wants to help me to correct my lifestyle and to rebalance my energies.

HEART OPENING

I now put my right hand on my heart.

HEALING MANTRA

"I am sending all my gratitude to (BOP's name), who is the messenger of the Cosmos and who has accepted to sacrifice himself to deliver the painful message.

I am also sending all my gratitude to the Cosmos, which loves me and wants me to fix something in my life."

I stay attuned and wait until I feel that a deep gratitude is flowing from my heart to (BOP's name) and to the Cosmos.

All my being enjoys this infusion of love and this warm, emotional stream warming me up body and soul.

I am also relieved to understand why I am suffering: pain is a message of the Cosmos conveyed by the Body-in-pain. Pain has a meaning, and it is a meaning of hope, not of blind destruction.

Then I do **two evaluations**.

FRUSTRATION

My frustration level which was…on a scale from 0 to 10 is lower and is now…

PAIN/ DISCOMFORT

My pain or discomfort level which was…is also lower and is now…

For example, the new frustration might be 3 and the pain level also 3.

ASTRAL CLAPPING

To thank the healing forces of the cosmos, which have manifested themselves again by this improvement, **I gently clap my hands in gratitude** in a state of light emotional trance.

TALKING TERMS

The improvement obtained allows me to visualize a BOP even closer and more friendly to me. I can now **shake hands** with (BOP's name) while looking him straight in the eyes.

SHAPE SHIFTING

I observe possible changes: If BOP was very old, he will probably be younger now. If he was too young, lacking maturity, he will perhaps be older. His character might also be improved.

EMOTIONAL WORK REVIEW

My view of suffering is considerably modified. **Pain is not just a nuisance, it is paradoxically, a friendly warning message.**

(BOP's name) is not an executioner or a trouble maker. He is a whistle blower informing me that the Cosmos are supporting me and want me to change for my own good.

I feel full of gratitude for (BOP's name) and for the Cosmos.

My faith in the Happy Healing Method is increasing. I am so happy to be able to guide my self-healing with positive results.

Phase 3. Humility And Asking For Forgiveness

STATEMENT

I realize that (BOP's name) has done **not one, but two sacrifices** to rescue me.

The first sacrifice is to accept to carry the message of physical pain.

The second sacrifice is an emotional and moral sacrifice.

In my selfishness, I ignored the pain experienced by (BOP's name), and I rejected him as a troublemaker and a traitor.

(BOP's name) was suffering from this emotional rejection even more than from the physical pain.

I imagine a single mother raising a child alone, sacrificing time, money, effort, and her private life for her child. At the end, I imagine the child completely ungrateful, accusing her mother of not supporting her as well as other mothers. Then the mother feels not only **ignored, but rejected, though she has done** so much for her child.

Until now, I was like the heartless child rejecting the loving mother.

"I realize how self centered I was and feel quite humbled. I beg (BOP's name) to forgive me. I commit myself to changing my attitude from now on to fully understand and support (BOP's name)."

HEART OPENING

I now put my right hand on my heart.

HEALING MANTRA

"I am ashamed of myself and I ask (BOP's name) to forgive my past attitude of rejection. I feel deeply humble and purified by the forgiveness of (BOP's name). I feel a new connection to (BOP's name). With this new start, I feel full of energy."

Then I do **two evaluations**.

FRUSTRATION

My frustration level which was….on a scale from 0 to 10 is lower and is now…

PAIN/ DISCOMFORT

My pain or discomfort level which was….is also lower and is now….

For example, the frustration could be now 0, and the pain still 2. After a quick decrease during phases 1 and 2, the pain level is not so easy to reduce. A residual pain remains.

It is also possible that the feelings towards BOP are now positive, for instance 3 on the positive scale, corresponding to rising sympathy for BOP.

ASTRAL CLAPPING

To thank the healing forces of the cosmos, which have manifested themselves by this improvement, **I gently clap in gratitude** in a state of light emotional trance.

TALKING TERMS

This new improvement allows me now to **hug BOP warmly**.

SHAPE SHIFTING

I observe possible changes: If BOP was very old, he will probably be younger now. If he was too young, lacking maturity, he will perhaps be older. His character might also be improved.

EMOTIONAL WORK REVIEW

My perspective is completely reversed during this emotional U-turn.

I started by recognizing the suffering of BOP (phase A) and felt a new empathy for BOP as a person, whom I named in phase B. This connection allowed me to analyze my feelings towards BOP and vice versa, feeling which were negative at the beginning.

Then with the compassion of phase 1, I realized that BOP was also a victim, and a victim who sacrificed a first time physically (Gratitude of phase 2) and a second time emotionally (Humility of phase 3). During this last phase, I realized that the one really to pity was not me but BOP, this suffering sentient being.

If there is "a bad guy," it is not BOP, it is me!

Until now, there has been a tragic misunderstanding. I was my own enemy. BOP was not my enemy, but my friend.

This discovery is like an emotional Big Bang, generating a deep transformation of my attitude and triggering a strong healing process.

This adjustment has created in me a powerful need and wish to support BOP. This desire sets up a completely **new healing field of energy.**

I experience **an emotional rebirth, full of hope for my health, physical, emotional, and spiritual.** Humility has helped me to grow spiritually.

My eyes can now see more clearly, my ears can now listen better, and my heart is now more open: I can now better speak with (BOP's name) and the Cosmos.

I will change. The keywords connected with re-birth are purification, simplification, elevation, and empowerment.

I will listen more to the divine presence, I will respect more the Law of Nature, I will be more one with the Cosmos.

Thank you, Cosmos! (or as appropriate for everyone: Thank you Universe, thank you God, thank you…).

Thank you also Happy Healing Process for taking me through this emotional discovery and transformation.

CYCLE OF POSITIVE FEELING

The previous cycle of negative feelings in 3 phases is now over. I enter now a **new cycle of 3 phases,** no longer of negative feelings, but of **positive feelings towards BOP. Huge difference producing a huge impact!**

The goal is no longer to reduce negativity, but to **increase positivity, which is much easier.**

Phase 4. Joy And Trust

STATEMENT

I realize that BOP and I form a team.

BOP cannot live without me, and I cannot live without BOP. We have to find a compromise and **enter into an agreement to live the best life possible together.**

We are a team. Like in a sports team, the team will win if the players play collectively, not anxious to make a personal show, but eager to **support the whole team.**

"(BOP's name) and I are both rowing in the same boat. I visualize (BOP's name) placed on the seat in front of me, and I row at the same rhythm as he rows, even though he is not as strong as I am because he is sick. Harmony is the key word.

Together, my life partner (BOP's name) and I are building our future with joy and trust. Incredible, (BOP's name) is no longer my worst enemy, but my best friend!

A rush of refreshing energy!"

HEART OPENING

I now put my right hand on my heart

HEALING MANTRA

"I feel the joy of forming a wonderful team with (BOP's name). We are rowing in the same boat with joy and mutual trust. We will win together, and the victory's name is good health."

BODY MAGNETIZATION

Now that I have entered the cycle of positive feelings for my body, **I can magnetize my Body-in-pain with the support of love.**

My right hand is still on my heart, transmitting my love to my whole body.

I now place **my left hand on the painful spot** (slightly above or with physical contact) **on the physical BOP,** and communicate to my body formerly in pain a new energy, **both a loving and magnetic energy.**

I exercise a double action, both emotional and physical, to help my body. With the **right hand on my heart,** I energize my body as a sentient being; with **my left hand on my painful spot**, I magnetize my body with vital energy.

Then I do **two evaluations**.

SYMPATHY (no more frustration, what a relief!)

My sympathy level which was….on a scale from 0 to 10 is higher and is now…

PAIN/ DISCOMFORT

My pain or discomfort level which was….is lower and is now…

For example', the positive feeling of sympathy was 3 and now could be 5 or 7. Sympathy is now love (above level 5, "sympathy" is "love").

The pain level is minimal, but still 0.5.

This is already a great result compared to the original level 7.

ASTRAL CLAPPING

To thank the healing forces of the cosmos, which have manifested themselves by this new improvement, **I gently clap in gratitude** in a state of light emotional trance.

Since I entered the cycle of positive feelings, the cycle of joy and love, this astral clapping of cosmic gratitude resonates even more.

I prolong the astral clapping to create a more powerful wave of joyful and happy healing.

I realize now that pain is significantly relieved, if not gone. **The healing process is gaining great momentum.**

TALKING TERMS

I can again hug (BOP's name) and kiss him.

SHAPE SHIFTING

I observe possible changes: If BOP was very old, he will probably be younger now. If he was too young, lacking maturity, he will perhaps be older. His character might be also improved.

EMOTIONAL WORK REVIEW

I know already that (BOP's name) is not my enemy, but on the contrary, **my best friend** who made a double sacrifice to rescue me by giving me the pain warning signal.

In this phase 4, I can enjoy openly this new cooperation with (BOP's name), not only a friend, but **an everyday partner**.

Thank you, Cosmos (or as appropriate for everyone: Thank you Universe, thank you God, thank you…). **Thank you also Happy Healing for now taking me into the happiness zone.**

Phase 5. Fusional Love

I can enter this phase 5 only if my positive feeling is a level 5 or above (the love zone, not simply the sympathy zone).

Channeling the Higher Self can take place only thanks to the love vibrations.

If my sympathy is under 5, under the love level, I have to work again emotionally and do another session to try to reach this level 5. Otherwise, experience shows that the conscious inner dialogue with the Higher Self cannot really start.

STATEMENT

"I am now in a state of fusional love with (BOP's name).

BOP is me and I am BOP.

I will now ask (BOP's name) to give me at least two or three tips, the precious tips of the cosmos, of which (BOP's name) is the messenger."

HEART OPENING

I now put my right hand on my heart.

I feel immediately the loving warmth of the presence of (BOP's name).

HEALING MANTRA

"Dear (BOP's name), what should I do so that you and I get better and better together? Please give me a few tips that I can implement today. Which tips of the Cosmos are you giving me?"

Tip 1…, tip 2…, tip 3…, tip 4…

"The tips of the Cosmos are given to me by (BOP's name) as a special cosmic blessing. These tips are the HEALING PLAN given to me by the Cosmos."

These tips, detailed in chapter 11, are usually split into 8 archetypal categories: **re-centering, doing less, reconnection with nature, physical activity, diet, sleep, artistic expression, social contacts.**

The most common tip to be given is the following in the re-centering category:

"Take 30 minutes per day just for yourself, to read, to listen to music, or to meditate."

The most powerful solution is always extremely simple: **the daily Sacred Break.**

BODY MAGNETIZATION

I can magnetize my body-in-pain as in phase 4, since now I am loving myself and my body, which is no longer in pain.

My right hand is still on my heart, transmitting my love to my whole body.

I now place **my left hand on the painful spot** (slightly above or with physical contact), **on the physical BOP**, and communicate to my body formerly in pain a new energy, **both a loving and magnetic energy.**

I exercise a double action, both emotional and physical, to help my body. With the **right hand on my heart**, I energize my body as a sentient being; with **my left hand on my painful spot**, I magnetize my body with vital energy.

Then I do **two evaluations**.

LOVE

My love level for (BOP's name) was already high and now reaches 9 or 10.

PAIN/ DISCOMFORT

My pain or discomfort level, which was nearly on zero (0.5), is now probably reaching zero.

ASTRAL CLAPPING

To thank the healing forces of the Cosmos, which have manifested themselves by this communication with my higher self, **I gently clap in gratitude** in a state of light emotional trance.

TALKING TERMS

I am now one with (BOP's name). We are not separated. We communicate instantly through a spiritual telepathy.

SHAPE SHIFTING

Very often, in this phase, I no longer perceive BOP as separate. We are one in this fusional love feeling. So to speak, I re-incorporate (BOP's name)!

EMOTIONAL WORK REVIEW

In this phase 5, a new goal has appeared.

As in the other phases, the goal was to **increase positive feelings and reduce pain**. But now, thanks to the high level of positivity which has been reached, the message of the Cosmos becomes more and more clear. My new goal is to understand it.

This Love for my body, which was in pain, but which is now pain free or nearly pain free, is already fulfilling the Cosmos's wishes.

I can now decipher the Cosmos's message: what needs to be changed in my values, lifestyle, habits, daily routine, so that the Cosmos no longer need to send a painful warning signal?

Through the 3 or 4 tips, the Cosmos is answering, as an oracle, the question that I put to (BOP's name). **These Tips of the Cosmos are a healing plan for me.**

This **cosmic coaching** is the most powerful coaching possible, emanating not from an external human coach, but from the inner voice of **the Higher Self**. Those tips are more genuine and to the point than if they were offered by a human coach. They have a strong motivational effect and will be better remembered.

Phase 6. Peace And Liberation

Phase 5 was reachable only with a sympathy/love level of 5 and above on a scale between 0 and 10.

To reach phase 6, the last phase, **a sympathy/ love level of 9 or 10 is recommended**. Love is the spiritual fuel which allows one to go further on higher spiritual planes.

STATEMENT

"I realize that through the process of Happy Healing, **I transform myself on an emotional and spiritual level.**

My feelings for my body are now positive. I am growing spiritually, becoming **less self-centered, and opening my heart more**.

I am filled with Love, Light, and physical well being.

My core values are influenced. As many survivors who have healed from a dreadful disease, **I value even more than before good human relationships and personal balance**. Money is only a goal among many."

HEART OPENING

I now put my right hand on my heart.

HEALING MANTRA

"I feel immediately the loving warmth of the presence of (BOP's name) and also the infinite presence of the Cosmos.

In this new state of well being with little pain, if any, I listen now not only to my body, which is no longer in pain, but also to my general environment.

I feel engulfed in an ocean of peace and of compassion.

The energy comes from nowhere and is everywhere: in me, in my body, in my environment, in the Cosmos.

I feel one with this peaceful emptiness which calms all my desires.

All my worries, may they be physical or emotional, are melting down.

I feel like floating; liberated, healed and happy."

SHORT HEALING MANTRA

**"I love my body and my body loves me.
I love the Cosmos and the Cosmos loves me.
I love myself and my higher self loves me."**

These two mantras can be repeated a few times in a powerful healing meditation.

ASTRAL CLAPPING

I conclude this last phase of Happy Healing with a long, long, **long astral clapping** as if I were gliding on a sacred lake of peaceful water, full of cosmic gratitude.

EMOTIONAL WORK REVIEW

Layer after layer, phase after phase, I practiced quite a few wonderful techniques.

- putting myself in the shoes of my Body-in-pain
- talking with my Body-in-pain, personalized with a name
- recycling negative feelings into positive ones
- interacting with my body, my heart, and my soul
- operating the astral representation of my physical body within the chamber of my heart

A great liberation was waiting for me at the end of the process.

I feel ONE with the FLOW and the ENERGY of the ONE!

CHAPTER 16

Recommendations After A Self-Healing Session

Should I go through the whole protocol?

Congratulations! You have been through the Happy Healing Protocol, perhaps only through the phases 1 and 2 if you were experiencing the method for the first time.

Hopefully, you feel better.

To go further: try to go through the protocol until phase 5 to obtain the healing plan of the Tips of the Cosmos.

If you are in the love zone and experiencing positive feelings at 8-10, you can surrender, let it go, and experience unconditional love in phase 6. If your goal is not only pain relief but also to start a healing process to heal from a dangerous disease, try to go also to the last phase, the phase 6, about a new philosophy of life.

Should I repeat sessions with the same BOP?

You can repeat with the same part of your Body-in-pain, BOP, as many times as you want.

You can choose the same BOP and change the name and the description of phase B.

Or you can keep the same name.

Just watch possible shape shifting (age, appearance, feelings). Your Body-in-pain, this sentient being, may react differently each time depending on the healing results you obtain.

Should I really report what is happening during the 8 steps?

Do not skip the reporting part: always write down with a pen your results. It will ground you and help you to go deeper during your session.

After a session, read your notes and complete them with specific comments which might come to your mind.

Important: by so doing, you will also document your health history and be more in charge of your health.

You are now taking your health into your owns hands. You became your own best health expert (and free of charge!). Congratulations on this fundamental self-empowerment!

Highly recommended: keep a health diary, where you will note your daily progresses, and the different reports on your Happy Healing sessions.

Should I do other sessions with another BOP?

You can also choose another Body Part, another BOP. The record is held by a patient who practiced Happy Healing for 12 BOPS successively!

You will discover so many fascinating things about your body.

The healing plan of the Tips of the Cosmos

The phase 5, "Tips of the Cosmos", is a gold mine of basic but powerful information given by your Higher Self, a very gifted invisible coach.

Write them down, but more than that: perform these tips! Action! Knock at the door, and the door will open. Do the prescribed exercises, and the Cosmos will do the follow-up.

Keep talking with your body after the session

Do not forget to practice this form of self-talk, talking with your BOP, especially each day during the first three days after your self-healing session. Anchor the Ritual until it becomes easy Routine. Then it will work for you, even if you do not think consciously about it.

Keep studying

Read and re-read the book *Happy Healing*. Re-read from time to time your notes and your diary.

Start helping others with the Happy Healing protocol

Try to help your relatives, friends, or colleagues who are in pain by sharing with them this self-healing philosophy and by walking them through the Happy Healing process.

Stay motivated on this pilgrimage of Happy Healing

Be happy with small results at the beginning.

Do it again and again, don't be discouraged.

Do astral clappings quite often to thank your Body-in-pain, to thank the Cosmos, to thank your Higher Self and your unconscious mind.

Believe in your wonderful self-healing potential

You will find out based on your own experience how to adjust the technique to your specific health problems, from the high level pain to the faintest nuance of discomfort.

Each time, you will be astonished at your psychosomatic reactivity and creativity! Your body will love it.

May all the Bodies-in-pain be happy again.

Happy Healing, dear reader, Happy Healing to you!

CHAPTER 17

The Success Formula for Happy Healing and The Love Message

The Happy Healing Success Formula

Let us review what to study, what to do and what to believe to optimize the chances of starting a powerful and successful healing process.

I call this **the Happy Healing Success Formula**, consisting in **9 important points.**

The 9 points Success Formula for Happy Healing:

1. Study the method and its philosophy

2. Cultivate the right healing attitude

3. Trust the Happy Healing process

4. Carefully prepare the healing equation

5. Meditate on the flying carpet of heart opening

6. Channel the healing plan: the Tips of the Cosmos

7. Document the session with the reporting and consultation forms and a diary

8.   Keep talking with the Body-in-pain after the session

9.   Apply the healing plan

Self-healing is in your power; the Success Formula reviews the work that enables you to self-heal - before a self-healing session, during a session, and after a session.

Before The Session

Point 1: Study the method and its philosophy

Before going through the self-healing protocol, it is recommended to study the Happy Healing method.

Get familiar with the compassionate philosophy of Happy Healing and the techniques which will guide you to a successful and happy self-healing.

Point 2: Cultivate the right healing attitude

It is recommended to cultivate the right healing attitudes developed in the first chapters. Wish to heal, soft approach, "no resignation, but no aggressiveness," and trusting the way your body will respond to your new attitude.

Practice Happy Healing often, be happy with encouraging small results, start again, and take note in a diary of your healing evolution.

Point 3: Trust the Happy Healing process

Accept the different visualizations which will be proposed to trigger positive emotions.

It works if you commit yourself to following the instructions. Do not question the assumptions which will be submitted to you. Go through the protocol with self-confidence in your abilities and trust the process.

If Happy Healing does not work so well for you, do not criticize the method, but try again.

Be sure that you are making a wise investment in time and dedication in your own interest, in the interest of your body, of your mind, of your soul.

During The Session

Point 4: Carefully prepare the healing equation

The way to properly set up the healing equation relative to phases A and B has been detailed in Chapter 10.

When the evaluation is precise and well thought out, you are creating the right basis to develop a successful healing transformation.

Point 5: Meditate on the flying carpet of heart opening

The emotional transformation of Happy Healing is made through a succession of compassionate moments for your Body-in-pain: open your heart, and your body will heal.

Say the prayers of Chapter 8, pronounce the healing mantras of the protocol, and fly on the flying carpet of compassionate meditation!

Point 6: Channel the healing plan: the Tips of the Cosmos

If you manage to reach the love zone, you will be able to channel from your Higher Self a few Tips of the Cosmos specially adapted to your health situation (Chapter 11).

What a great reward! Just love yourself, and you will receive a readymade Healing Plan from the cosmic coach!

Point 7: Document the session with the reporting and consultation forms and a diary

Write down the pain/discomfort spots and zones found during the body scan on the consultation form.

For each of the 8 phases, write down the evolution of the different parameters on the reporting form.

After The Session

Point 8: Keep talking with the Body-in-pain after the session

After the session, it is important to keep talking with BOP, with the Body-in-pain, or the Body-once-in-pain.

You managed to communicate consciously with the emotional intelligence of your body. You want to activate, from time to time, this wonderful connection through which the healing process takes place. This is the precious link to the Cosmos's healing power!

Point 9: Apply the healing plan

If you had the chance to receive a few Tips of the Cosmos, you do not want to lose this huge benefit. Meditate regularly on these tips, note in your diary the progress you make thanks to the application of this healing plan.

Life is simple, but you must follow the right path. The healing plan is helping you to have a healthy and better life.

Since Happy Healing is about loving yourself, let us quote RUMI, the great Sufi master of the 13th century:

"Love is the cure,
for your pain will keep giving birth to more pain
until your eyes constantly exhale love
as effortlessly as your body yields its scent"

Until love is completely experienced as a physical sensation, as a fluid emanating from the eyes, as a scent emanating from the body, pain will nourish more pain, and healing is hindered.

With love, the cure will take place.
With love for your body, you will enjoy the zero pain option:
Love more and suffer less,
Love your Body-in-pain, and your pain and your discomfort will be relieved!

Conclusion

If there is a virtue that pain is teaching to the patient as well as to the therapist, it is humility.

Humility facing the psychosomatic disturbances and disorders, both unpleasant and mysterious…

With the self-healing protocol of Happy Healing, you hold in your hands a precious tool that can assist you in relieving pain and discomfort while starting a true healing process.

Does it always work? Does it systematically reduce your pain to zero?
With humility, I must say, no.

Does it often work, even if sometimes you have to repeat the protocol and go through it with not only one BOP, but two or three different BOPs?
With humility, I am happy to say, yes.

But it is your responsibility, your choice, your plan.
Happy Healing is a tool: you are the master craftsperson.

Healing is always possible at different levels. Even if in some cases you cannot heal much on the physical level, you can always heal on the emotional, mental, or spiritual level.

With humility, this is my last recommendation.

Appendix: Consultation & Reporting Forms

On the following pages, you will find blank copies of the Consultation and Reporting Forms. As introduced in Chapter 6, the Consultation and Reporting Forms are helpful tools to use as you begin self-healing with the Happy Healing Protocol.

These forms will allow you to identify your BOPs and keep track of your progress as your work through the phases towards becoming pain free. I encourage you to make copies of these forms and use them for all of your self-healing sessions.

As you begin to use Happy Healing, you may want to start by using the much shorter 4 step version of the protocol. It is a wonderful way to familiarize yourself with the protocol and your own healing.

Visit **www.HappyHealingBook.com/bonus** to receive your copy of this bonus mini-protocol.

HAPPY HEALING

Consultation Form

Patient's name:____

Date of birth　　:_____________________　　Telephone　:________________

E-Mail　　　　　:_____________________　　Occupation:________________

Session　　　　:_____________________　　Date　　　　:________________

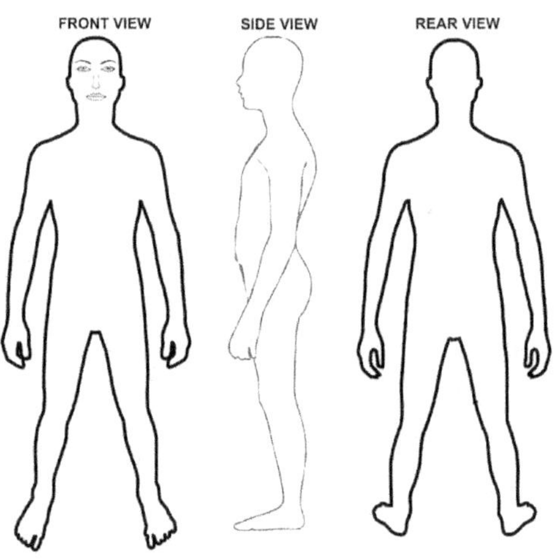

BOP's LOCATION (BOP = Body Part in Pain)

The body scan for pain and discomfort* spots and zones

BOP #1 is...

***DISCOMFORT CHECKLIST**

STAGNATION
Low energy, slow circulation, numbness, cold, blockage,
restriction, muscular weakness, loss of control,
feeling overwhelmed

BLOCKAGE WITH PRESSURE
heaviness, hardness, pressure, tension, STRESS
STOP AND GO
tickling, cramping, shaking, shivering, convulsion, pulsation, beats
RUSH
itching, burning, hot, radiation

HAPPY HEALING
REPORTING FORM
Phases A + B and phases 1 to 6

Name:

Date:

Session:

EVALUATION PHASES A and B

PHASE A. BODY SCAN

1. Identifying the #1 Body Part(**BOP**) in pain or discomfort

....

2. Grade on scale between 0 and 10 the **pain / discomfort level** ....

PHASE B. NAMING BOP and FRUSTRATION EVALUATION

1. Give a **name** to the Body-Part-in-pain BOP as a male/female person ....

....

2. Find out the age.................of BOP, and his/her **eyes**...................... and
   hair.......................... **color.**
3. Grade between 0 and 10 your **level of frustration / guilt** ....
   towards...................(BOP's name)
4. Evaluate the **distance** between you and (BOP's name)....................................

TRANSFORMATION PHASES 1 to 6

	MENTAL IMAGE	EMOTION	HATE*	LOVE*	PAIN*
PHASE1	co-victim totally in the boiling pot	compassion			
PHASE2	cosmos's messenger physical sacrifice	admiration gratefulness			
PHASE3	double sacrifice, physical/moral	humility asking for forgiveness			
PHASE4	companion teamplayer	joy & trust			
PHASE5	higher Self's voice	fusional love			
PHASE6	cosmic oneness	peacefulness			
COMMENTS:					

Hate* = negative feelings like frustration, anger, guilt, fear
Love* = positive feelings like sympathy and love
Pain* = pain or discomfort

HAPPY HEALING
Consultation Form

Patient's name:____

Date of birth   :___________________   Telephone :_______________

E-Mail   :___________________   Occupation:_______________

Session   :___________________   Date   :_______________

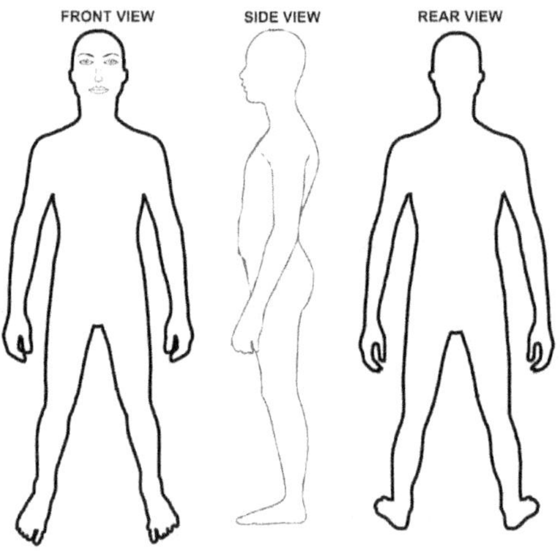

BOP's LOCATION (BOP = Body Part in Pain)
The body scan for pain and discomfort* spots and zones

BOP #1 is...

---

*DISCOMFORT CHECKLIST

STAGNATION
Low energy, slow circulation, numbness, cold, blockage, restriction, muscular weakness, loss of control, feeling overwhelmed

BLOCKAGE WITH PRESSURE
heaviness, hardness, pressure, tension, STRESS
STOP AND GO
tickling, cramping, shaking, shivering, convulsion, pulsation, beats
RUSH
itching, burning, hot, radiation

HAPPY HEALING
REPORTING FORM
Phases A + B and phases 1 to 6

Name:

Date:

Session:

EVALUATION PHASES A and B

PHASE A. BODY SCAN
1. Identifying the #1 Body Part(**BOP**) in pain or discomfort
....
2. Grade on scale between 0 and 10 the **pain / discomfort level** ....

PHASE B. NAMING BOP and FRUSTRATION EVALUATION
1. Give a **name** to the Body-Part-in-pain BOP as a male/female person ....
....
2. Find out the age.................of BOP, and his/her **eyes**...................... and
   hair............................ **color**.
3. Grade between 0 and 10 your **level of frustration / guilt** ....
   towards....................(BOP's name)
4. Evaluate the **distance** between you and (BOP's name)...................................

TRANSFORMATION PHASES 1 to 6

	MENTAL IMAGE	EMOTION	HATE*	LOVE*	PAIN*
PHASE1	co-victim totally in the boiling pot	compassion			
PHASE2	cosmos's messenger physical sacrifice	admiration gratefulness			
PHASE3	double sacrifice, physical/moral	humility asking for forgiveness			
PHASE4	companion teamplayer	joy & trust			
PHASE5	higher Self's voice	fusional love			
PHASE6	cosmic oneness	peacefulness			

COMMENTS:

Hate* = negative feelings like frustration, anger, guilt, fear
Love* = positive feelings like sympathy and love
Pain* = pain or discomfort

Acknowledgements

First of all, I would like to thank BOP.

Who is BOP?

BOP, the Body-part-in-pain, is our suffering partner when physical pain and discomfort are showing up.

I thank BOP, all the BOPs, suffering from pain, and also suffering from our irritation and frustration, for their endless patience.

I feel so grateful to the BOPs of all the patients I have treated who helped me to put together the healing protocol of Happy Healing.

This book will help the readers practice self-healing with this emotional and compassionate approach.

May all BOPS of patients be pain free and happy!

Writing and Publishing this self-healing method in English was not that easy for me, a Frenchman living in Germany.

Fortunately, I attended a workshop by Mike Koenigs and Ed Rush in California about self-publishing.

Thanks to Mike and Ed, I realized that self-publishing is as easy and rewarding as self-healing!

At this workshop and after this workshop, I had the opportunity to be coached by Rory Carruthers, author of many bestsellers and expert in self-publishing.

Thanks to his invaluable assistance, and to the precious and subtle editing of his wife, Carly, you can read Happy Healing…and apply it to boost your own health, and possibly help others do the same!

A huge thank you to you both, Carly and Rory, and to your team.

About The Author

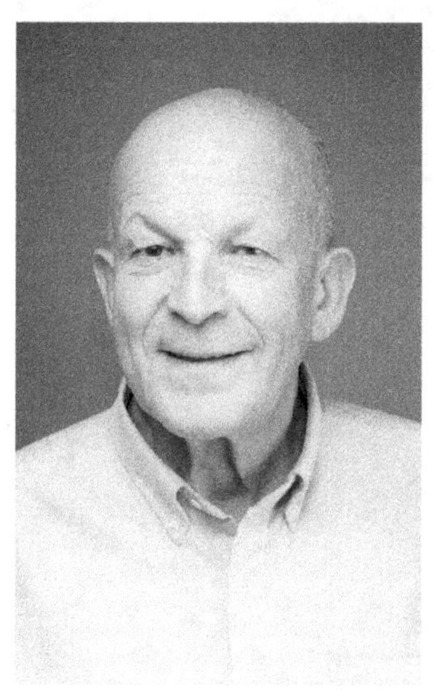

Dominique Bourlet became a therapist and a healer without planning it.

Part time horse whisperer nearly 20 years ago, he realized that horse whispering was, at the core, a therapy for horses, a manual therapy with specific massages, gestures, and body contacts. It was also a psychotherapy, helping horses overcome their fears and perceive trainers and riders as partners and not enemies.

This, and a new method to teach horse riding that he created, the Equestrian Mime Program, led him to study yoga and then Ayurveda, this traditional Indian medical system, in the south of India.

The incredible association between energetic massages and ancient medical and spiritual traditions, such as practiced in all Asia, was a mind-blowing experience.

In just a few years, he learned more than 20 manual therapies in 10 Asian countries, from India to Japan.

In 2009, he published in French *Prier Avec Les Guérisseurs Philippins*, a book explaining the work of the wonder healers of the Philippines.

He still spends a few weeks in Asia every year to "recharge" his healing batteries.

Dominique Bourlet became a German "Heilpraktiker," or alternative practitioner, in Berlin, Germany, in 2007.

For 12 years, he has been developing the Happy Healing emotional method to complement the physical approach of Chinese acupressure that he practices, as well as distant healing and spiritual healing.

Learn more at www.DomBourlet.com

www.ingramcontent.com/pod-product-compliance
Lightning Source LLC
LaVergne TN
LVHW020749200726
843506LV00009B/957